Nomad

**The Heart of the Matter: Cleaning and Fueling
the Body's Plumbing System**

NoMAD
The Heart of the Matter: Cleaning and Fueling the Body's
Plumbing System

What are the NoMAD Plans?

Developed by Dr Ash Kapoor, the NoMAD Plans represent a transformative approach to health and wellness that combines the wisdom of ancestral practices with contemporary medical insights. The name "NoMAD" not only suggests a journey through the intricate realm of health but also stands for its foundational principles: Nutritional Optimisation, Mindful Adaptation, and Detoxification.

At the heart of NoMAD is the 6R Framework—Restore, Release, Repair, Renew, Reframe, and Represent. This methodology addresses the root causes of illness, combats chronic inflammation, and cultivates authentic vitality, guiding individuals through a transformative process.

Tailored specifically to each individual, NoMAD journeys are meticulously crafted to rebalance the body, strengthen the mind, and rejuvenate overall health. By integrating ancestral practices with cutting-edge, innovative treatments—all under strict medical oversight—NoMAD Plans offer a personalised pathway to sustainable, long-lasting well-being that resonates with your unique life circumstances.

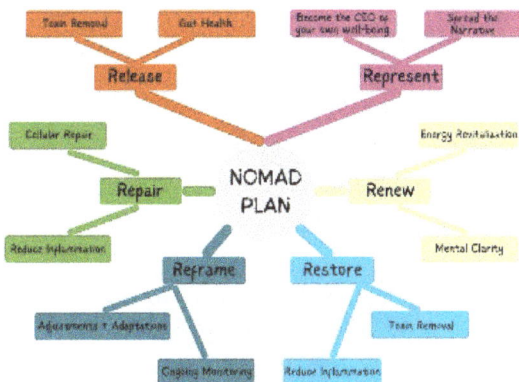

Levitas One:
"As Is In, As Is Out"

Reflecting the belief that our internal well-being is mirrored in our external environment. Founded by Dr. Ash Kapoor, Levitas One serves as the vehicle for delivering NoMAD's treatment plans. It envisions a healthcare future where patients are at the centre of a fully integrated, multidisciplinary approach. Guided by Nomads 6 Rs— Restore, Release, Repair, Renew, and Reframe, Represent— Levitas One empowers self-care through personalised guidance and minimal intervention, promoting long-term health, balance, and sustainability.

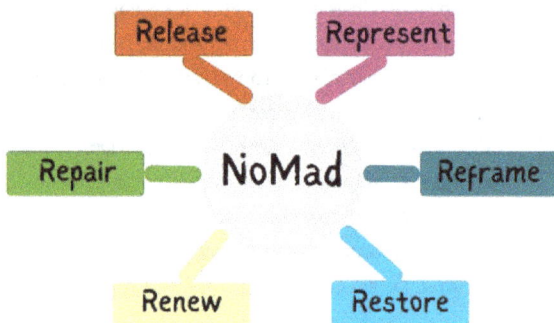

Contents

Preface

In almost 35 years of clinical practice, I have witnessed countless patients progress through the complex cycle of disease and treatment. It has often led me to reflect on what has truly been achieved in terms of quality of life. As healthcare professionals, we focus on managing symptoms, prescribing medications, and mitigating crises. But I have come to question whether, in our well-intentioned pursuit of managing disease, we may have missed the opportunity to intervene earlier—at a point where self-care and lifestyle changes could have altered the trajectory of illness altogether. Instead of waiting for the disease to escalate, could we have empowered patients to take control of their health to address the underlying inflammation and dysfunction that silently drive so many of these chronic conditions?

The lessons learned from these reflections have inspired the pages of this book. It is written not just as a guide for managing heart disease but as a broader exploration of how we can rethink cardiovascular health. This book aims to provide insights into a condition that becomes increasingly significant as we age, given its profound impact on our risk of mortality and morbidity. Heart disease is not just a clinical issue; **it is** a deeply personal concern that touches the lives of every patient and their families.

Through integrating non-pharmacological innovations, holistic strategies, and patient-centred care, I hope to offer a perspective that shifts the focus from merely treating disease to fostering health. This approach recognises that the body's innate ability to heal and adapt is often overlooked in favour of escalating medications. By acknowledging this potential, we can create a more compassionate and effective pathway to heart health.

May this book inspire readers to look beyond traditional boundaries, to consider a more comprehensive and integrative approach to cardiac care that embraces prevention, lifestyle, and self-empowerment as cornerstones of true well-being.

— *Dr. Ash Kapoor*

Chapter 1
Embracing a Holistic
Approach to Cardiac Care

Introduction

In today's rapidly evolving medical landscape, the approach to heart health is undergoing a profound transformation. Traditionally dominated by pharmaceutical interventions and invasive procedures, the paradigm is shifting towards a more holistic, preventive strategy that emphasises the power of lifestyle changes, dietary adjustments, and natural therapies. This shift is not merely a trend but a response to decades of research and clinical observations that highlight the critical role of everyday choices in the management and prevention of heart disease. With cardiovascular disease remaining the leading cause of death globally, this rethinking of cardiac care offers a beacon of hope for millions seeking not only to treat, but to truly heal and rejuvenate their heart health.

The Evolution of Cardiac Care: From Reactive to Proactive

Cardiac care has come a long way from the days when treatment options were limited to reactive interventions and surgical remedies. The discovery of cholesterol's role in heart disease, for instance, led to the development of statins, which have been a mainstay in heart disease prevention. Statins are undeniably effective in lowering cholesterol levels and have significantly reduced cardiovascular events in high-risk populations. However, despite their benefits, the conversation around statins and similar interventions has grown more nuanced. Increasing awareness of their limitations, potential side effects, and the over-reliance on pharmacological management alone has led to a critical reevaluation of how we approach heart disease.

Parallel to this, the field of cardiology has seen a burgeoning interest in understanding how non-pharmacological factors such as diet, exercise, psychological stress, and sleep influence heart health. This holistic view is supported by a growing body of evidence that lifestyle interventions can not only prevent, but, in some cases, reverse coronary artery disease. Landmark programs like the Ornish Lifestyle Medicine program have demonstrated that comprehensive lifestyle changes—incorporating a plant-based diet, regular physical activity, stress management techniques, and social support—can significantly improve cardiovascular health, potentially even leading to regression of atherosclerotic plaques. This evidence challenges the traditional model of treating symptoms rather than addressing root causes and has sparked a paradigm shift towards viewing the heart not as an isolated organ but as an integrated component of a complex, dynamic system.

Rethinking Risk: The Multifaceted Nature of Heart Disease

Heart disease is no longer seen as a condition driven solely by lipid imbalances or high blood pressure. The new understanding is that heart disease is a multifactorial condition, influenced by a range of biological, psychological, and environmental factors. Chronic inflammation, oxidative stress, insulin resistance, and hormonal imbalances all play a role in the development and progression of cardiac diseases. Emerging research is now revealing that these factors are highly responsive to changes in lifestyle, such as the adoption of an anti-inflammatory diet, stress reduction techniques, and improved sleep hygiene.

Moreover, psychosocial factors—such as depression, anxiety, social isolation, and job-related stress—are now recognised as significant contributors to cardiovascular risk. This broader perspective underscores the importance of addressing mental and emotional well-being as part of a comprehensive approach to heart health. Patients and practitioners alike are realising that true heart health cannot be achieved through medication alone but requires a nuanced approach that fosters well-being at multiple levels: physical, mental, and emotional.

Embracing a Preventive Mindset: The Role of Diet and Lifestyle

The modern approach to heart health advocates for a preventive mindset, where dietary and lifestyle modifications are prioritised from an early age to promote long-term cardiovascular health. Plant-based diets, for example, have been shown to lower blood pressure, improve cholesterol profiles, and reduce systemic inflammation, all of which contribute to lower rates of heart disease. Incorporating foods rich in antioxidants, polyphenols, and essential fatty acids—such as leafy greens, berries, nuts, and fatty fish—can significantly enhance heart health by reducing oxidative stress and enhancing endothelial function.

Regular physical activity, meanwhile, not only strengthens the heart muscle but also improves blood pressure, glucose metabolism, and lipid profiles. Activities that promote cardiovascular fitness—such as aerobic exercises, yoga, and high-intensity interval training—are crucial components of a heart-healthy lifestyle. Additionally, the value of mind-body practices like mindfulness meditation and yoga, which have been shown to reduce stress and lower blood pressure, is gaining recognition as an integral part of holistic cardiac care.

The Growing Importance of Natural Therapies and Herbal Medicines

As we gain deeper insights into the biological processes that underlie heart conditions, the role of natural and lifestyle-based therapies has become increasingly prominent. Dietary adjustments, for example, can modulate inflammatory processes that are central to the development of atherosclerosis. Similarly, regular physical activity is known to improve blood pressure and glucose metabolism, reducing the risk of heart disease. Natural substances like omega-3 fatty acids, coenzyme Q_{10}, magnesium, and green tea extract are being studied for their potential cardioprotective effects, offering patients alternatives that complement traditional medical treatments.

Additionally, there is a resurgence of interest in herbal supplements, which have been used for centuries in traditional medicine systems. Hawthorn, for instance, is revered in both Western herbalism and traditional Chinese medicine for its ability to strengthen the heart, lower blood pressure, and improve circulation. Similarly, turmeric, with its potent anti-inflammatory and antioxidant properties, has shown promise in preventing atherosclerosis and improving overall cardiovascular health. These natural therapies, often used in combination with conventional treatments, can offer a more balanced and less invasive approach to managing heart disease.

Personalised Medicine: The Future of Cardiac Care

Another frontier in modern cardiology is the movement towards personalised medicine. Genetic testing, advanced imaging techniques, and biomarker analysis are enabling clinicians to tailor treatments to the individual, considering factors such as genetic predispositions, unique metabolic profiles, and environmental influences. This level of customisation allows for more precise interventions, reducing the risk of adverse effects and enhancing treatment efficacy. Personalised medicine also aligns seamlessly with holistic approaches, as it considers the patient's entire health profile rather than focusing on isolated symptoms.

A Call to Action: Empowering Patients Through Knowledge and Choice

This book seeks to redefine how we view and approach heart disease. It is not just about managing symptoms or preventing complications; it is about empowering patients with knowledge and giving them the tools to take control of their heart health in a more natural, sustainable way. Each chapter will delve into specific aspects of holistic cardiac care, from the science behind dietary impacts on heart health to the latest research on non-pharmacological interventions. By the end of this book, readers will have a comprehensive understanding of how a holistic approach can not only complement traditional cardiac care but often provide a preferable alternative, guiding them towards long-term health and vitality.

This new way of thinking about cardiac care is not just a medical revolution—it is a movement towards true wellness, where the heart is seen as both a physical and emotional centre, responsive to love, stress, and everything in between. As science continues to reveal the intricate connections between lifestyle and heart health, the path forward becomes clear: a preventive, holistic approach is not just an option but a necessity in the fight against heart disease.

Summary: Embracing a Holistic Approach to Cardiac Care

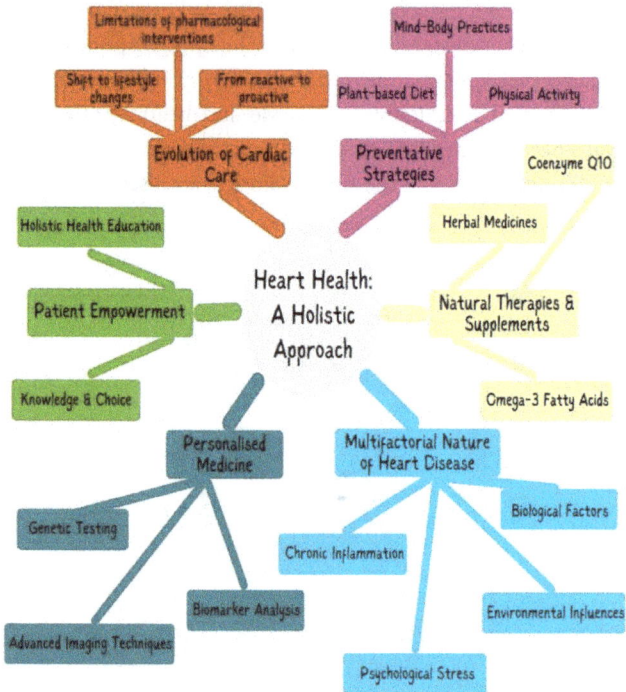

Chapter 2
The Role of Statins in Managing Coronary Artery Disease

Introduction

The widespread prescription of statins has reshaped the landscape of cardiovascular disease management. Positioned as a primary defence against heart disease, this chapter reevaluates the efficacy and implications of statin therapy, emphasising the importance of understanding both its benefits and limitations. The focus of this chapter extends beyond statins themselves, considering the broader mechanisms at play in heart disease, particularly the role of inflammation—a concept that has gained significant traction in the last few decades. This chapter will delve into why inflammation is increasingly seen as a key driver of cardiovascular disease and why addressing it is critical, rather than relying solely on pharmaceutical interventions or invasive procedures.

Understanding Statins

Statins inhibit the enzyme HMG-CoA reductase in the liver, crucial for cholesterol production. By reducing low-density lipoprotein (LDL) cholesterol, statins are believed to decrease the risk of heart attacks and strokes. However, the mechanism by which LDL reduction translates to cardiovascular benefit is more complex than initially thought. While high LDL levels are associated with an increased risk of coronary artery disease (CAD), simply lowering cholesterol without addressing underlying inflammatory processes may not provide comprehensive protection against heart disease. This raises the question of whether cholesterol management alone is sufficient or if a more nuanced approach—targeting inflammation—is necessary for optimal cardiovascular health.

Inflammation: The Hidden Culprit in Heart Disease

In recent years, researchers have begun to recognise that inflammation, not just lipid levels, plays a critical role in the pathogenesis of coronary artery disease. Studies such as the Canakinumab Anti-inflammatory Thrombosis Outcome Study (CANTOS) trial have shifted the spotlight towards inflammation as a therapeutic target. The CANTOS trial, conducted by Ridker et al. (2017), investigated the effect of canakinumab, an anti-inflammatory drug, on cardiovascular outcomes in patients with a history of heart attacks. The study found that targeting inflammation independent of lipid levels led to a significant reduction in recurrent cardiovascular events, thus validating the inflammatory hypothesis of heart disease.

This landmark trial demonstrated that patients receiving canakinumab had a 15% reduction in the risk of recurrent heart attacks, independent of any change in cholesterol levels. The results highlighted that inflammation, rather than cholesterol alone, is a major driver of atherosclerosis progression. It was the first major clinical trial to prove that lowering inflammation could reduce cardiovascular risk, even without changes in LDL cholesterol levels.

Mechanisms Linking Inflammation to Atherosclerosis

The underlying mechanisms linking inflammation to coronary artery disease involve complex interactions between the immune system and vascular tissues. Atherosclerosis, once considered a passive accumulation of lipids within the arterial walls, is now understood to be a dynamic inflammatory process. LDL particles that infiltrate the arterial walls undergo oxidation, triggering an immune response. This response recruits monocytes and macrophages, which engulf the oxidised LDL, forming foam cells that contribute to plaque buildup.

Pro-inflammatory cytokines like interleukin-1 (IL-1), tumour necrosis factor-alpha (TNF-α), and interleukin-6 (IL-6) are released, perpetuating a cycle of inflammation that destabilises plaques and makes them more likely to rupture. Plaque rupture, in turn, leads to thrombus formation, the immediate cause of most heart attacks. Therefore, addressing inflammation at its root may not only prevent plaque formation but also reduce the likelihood of acute coronary events.

Why Inflammation Matters More Than Cholesterol

Given the pivotal role of inflammation in heart disease, focusing solely on cholesterol management might overlook the root cause of atherosclerosis. Statins do have anti-inflammatory properties, which may account for a portion of their cardiovascular benefits. For instance, statins reduce C-reactive protein (CRP), a marker of inflammation, suggesting that their benefit extends beyond mere cholesterol reduction. However, the question remains whether other strategies could more directly and effectively address the inflammatory component of heart disease.

Statins and Inflammation: A Double-Edged Sword?

While statins have anti-inflammatory effects, their use is not without drawbacks. A study by Mansi et al. (2018) found that chronic statin use may impair muscle function, potentially leading to exercise intolerance, which paradoxically could reduce the cardiovascular benefits of physical activity. This highlights the need for approaches that enhance, rather than compromise, a patient's capacity to engage in heart-healthy behaviours.

Moreover, a study by Bruckert et al. (2005) indicated that muscle symptoms like myopathy and rhabdomyolysis, though rare, are more prevalent among statin users. This risk, albeit low, can lead to a reduction in exercise adherence due to discomfort, which is counterproductive in the broader context of cardiovascular health. If muscle symptoms deter patients from physical activity—a cornerstone of heart disease prevention—then the overall benefit of statin therapy may be diminished.

Reevaluating Risk: Inflammation as a Target for Therapy

Given the growing body of evidence implicating inflammation as a central driver of heart disease, therapeutic strategies that directly target inflammatory pathways are gaining attention. For example, colchicine, an anti-inflammatory drug traditionally used for gout, has shown promise in reducing cardiovascular events. The LoDoCo2 trial (Nidorf et al., 2020) demonstrated that low-dose colchicine significantly reduced the incidence of major adverse cardiovascular events in patients with chronic coronary disease, further supporting the role of inflammation in heart disease progression.

In another study, Tardif et al. (2019) investigated the use of colchicine in patients who had recently suffered a heart attack. The COLCOT trial found that colchicine reduced the risk of stroke and coronary revascularisation by 34%, reinforcing the concept that inflammation reduction is an effective strategy for cardiovascular event prevention.

Beyond Statins: Integrative Approaches to Lower Inflammation

The emphasis on inflammation as a therapeutic target opens the door to various non-pharmacological strategies. Lifestyle interventions that include dietary modifications, regular physical activity, and stress management techniques have been shown to reduce systemic inflammation. The Mediterranean diet, rich in anti-inflammatory compounds like omega-3 fatty acids, polyphenols, and fibre, has been associated with lower CRP levels and reduced cardiovascular risk (Estruch et al., 2018). Similarly, the DASH diet (Dietary Approaches to Stop Hypertension) has been shown to lower blood pressure and reduce systemic inflammation.

Moreover, mind-body interventions like yoga and meditation, which reduce stress—a key contributor to inflammation—are increasingly recognised as valuable components of holistic cardiac care. A study by Lavretsky et al. (2013) found that yoga and meditation significantly reduced inflammatory markers and improved heart rate variability, an indicator of autonomic nervous system balance, which is linked to better cardiovascular outcomes.

Limitations of the Conventional Approach: Why Lifestyle Matters

The traditional focus on cholesterol reduction has led to an over-reliance on statins and other lipid-lowering therapies, often at the expense of addressing other modifiable risk factors like diet, exercise, and stress. While statins are effective in reducing LDL cholesterol, they do not fully address the multifactorial nature of heart disease. For example, a person with low cholesterol but high levels of CRP or IL-6 is still at significant risk of a cardiovascular event due to underlying inflammation.

Furthermore, lifestyle interventions have shown effects comparable to or exceeding those of pharmacological therapies in certain populations. The Lyon Diet Heart Study (de Lorgeril et al., 1999) found that adherence to a Mediterranean diet reduced cardiovascular events by 70%—a reduction greater than that achieved by most cholesterol-lowering medications. This underscores the potential for lifestyle changes to not only complement but, in some cases, surpass pharmacological interventions in effectiveness.

Conclusion

The reliance on pharmaceutical interventions and surgical procedures as the primary means of managing heart disease is gradually giving way to a more comprehensive, holistic approach that prioritises inflammation reduction, lifestyle modifications, and Personalised medicine. As evidence continues to mount, it is clear that inflammation plays a more critical role in heart disease than previously acknowledged, necessitating a shift in both clinical practice and patient education.

While statins will continue to be an essential tool in the cardiologist's armamentarium, their role should be seen as part of a broader strategy that encompasses dietary changes, physical activity, stress reduction, and other anti-inflammatory approaches. By shifting the focus towards a more integrative, inflammation-centred view of heart disease, we can hope to achieve better outcomes, reduce the burden of cardiovascular disease, and empower patients to take control of their heart health in a more meaningful and sustainable way.

Summary: The Role of Statins in Managing Coronary Artery Disease

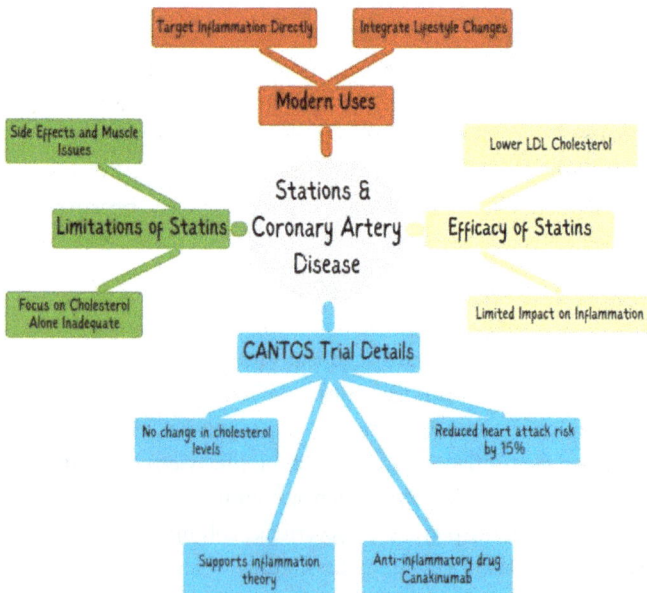

Chapter 3
Lifestyle Approaches to Managing Coronary Artery Disease

Introduction

As our understanding of coronary artery disease (CAD) evolves, the role of non-pharmacological interventions has become increasingly prominent. Once seen as mere adjuncts to pharmaceutical management, lifestyle modifications are now recognised as foundational strategies in both the prevention and management of CAD. These interventions can significantly alter the course of the disease, potentially reducing or even eliminating the need for medications like statins. This chapter explores how lifestyle changes, including diet, exercise, stress management, and other holistic approaches, target the root causes of CAD—namely, inflammation, oxidative stress, and endothelial dysfunction. By addressing these underlying factors, lifestyle modifications can profoundly influence heart health, offering a more sustainable and empowering approach to disease management.

The Pathophysiology of CAD

The development of CAD is deeply entwined with inflammatory processes, which go beyond simple cholesterol accumulation. Inflammation, immune system involvement, oxidative stress, and endothelial dysfunction contribute to the formation of arterial plaques that can rupture, leading to serious cardiovascular events such as heart attacks and strokes. This complex interplay underscores the potential of lifestyle changes to influence fundamental disease mechanisms. Unlike pharmacological treatments that often target symptoms or specific pathways, lifestyle interventions can act more comprehensively, addressing the root causes of inflammation and promoting overall cardiovascular health.

Dietary Influence on CAD

Nutritional Impact

Diet is one of the most influential factors in cardiovascular health. Diets rich in antioxidants and low in processed foods can modulate the body's inflammatory response. The Mediterranean and DASH (Dietary Approaches to Stop Hypertension) diets, rich in fruits, vegetables, whole grains, and lean proteins, have been clinically shown to reduce the incidence of major cardiovascular events. These diets provide essential nutrients that support heart health, stabilise blood vessels, and reduce inflammation, all of which are crucial in preventing CAD progression.

The anti-inflammatory properties of foods such as nuts, seeds, fatty fish, and olive oil are well-documented. Omega-3 fatty acids, found abundantly in fatty fish like salmon and in plant-based sources such as flaxseeds and chia seeds, are particularly noteworthy. Omega-3s help reduce the risk of plaque formation and heart disease by modulating inflammatory pathways, decreasing triglyceride levels, and improving endothelial function. These benefits are further supported by evidence showing that individuals who consume diets high in omega-3s have a lower incidence of cardiovascular events compared to those following a standard Western diet.

Scientific Evidence

A comprehensive study published in the *Journal of the American College of Cardiology* highlighted that individuals adhering to the Mediterranean diet showed a significant reduction in cardiovascular risk factors, including lower levels of CRP (C-reactive protein), a marker of inflammation, and improved overall heart health compared to those following a standard Western diet (Estruch et al., 2018). Another study found that the DASH diet led to significant reductions in both systolic and diastolic blood pressure, contributing to decreased CAD risk (Appel et al., 1997). These findings underscore the importance of dietary choices in modulating inflammation and reducing cardiovascular risk.

Physical Activity and Heart Health

Benefits of Exercise

Regular physical activity is another critical component of lifestyle management for CAD. Exercise enhances endothelial function, lowers blood pressure, and improves lipid profiles, all of which contribute to better cardiovascular outcomes. Activities such as walking, cycling, and swimming are particularly beneficial for maintaining cardiovascular health. Exercise also promotes weight management, reduces insulin resistance, and decreases inflammation, creating a cascade of positive effects that reduce CAD risk.

Engaging in aerobic exercise, such as brisk walking or cycling, has been shown to lower markers of inflammation, such as CRP and IL-6, while also increasing levels of anti-inflammatory cytokines like IL-10. This balance helps reduce the overall inflammatory burden on the cardiovascular system. Resistance training, on the other hand, can improve muscle strength and glucose metabolism, further supporting heart health.

Clinical Support

Research published in *Circulation* found that moderate to vigorous exercise reduces the risk of endothelial dysfunction and subsequently lowers the incidence of CAD (Lavie et al., 2019). The study emphasised that even short bouts of exercise could have significant benefits, particularly when performed consistently over time. These findings are reinforced by meta-analyses showing that regular physical activity is associated with a 30% reduction in the risk of developing cardiovascular disease (Anderson et al., 2016).

Stress Management and Cardiovascular Risk

Link Between Stress and Heart Health

Chronic stress has a profound impact on cardiovascular health. Stress influences the heart through direct mechanisms such as increased blood pressure and hormonal fluctuations, which contribute to heart disease. It can also exacerbate inflammation, leading to endothelial dysfunction and promoting atherosclerosis. Addressing stress is, therefore, a crucial component of holistic cardiac care.

Stress Reduction Techniques

Mindfulness, yoga, and regular physical exercise can significantly reduce stress levels and, by extension, improve cardiovascular health. These practices reduce levels of cortisol, a stress hormone that can increase blood pressure and promote inflammatory processes. Programs integrating mindfulness and yoga have been shown to decrease both physiological and psychological stress markers in cardiac patients, leading to better outcomes.

A study published in *Journal of Behavioural Medicine* found that mindfulness-based stress reduction (MBSR) significantly lowered CRP levels and improved heart rate variability (HRV), both of which are indicators of improved cardiovascular health (Burg et al., 2019). This suggests that mind-body practices can play a pivotal role in managing CAD, especially for patients who experience high levels of stress or anxiety.

Case Studies and Clinical Evidence

Real-Life Success Stories

Detailed narratives of individuals who have reversed or managed their CAD through lifestyle interventions provide compelling evidence of the efficacy of these approaches. One case study described a 52-year-old male patient with significant CAD who, after adopting comprehensive lifestyle changes including a plant-based diet, regular physical activity, and stress management techniques, experienced improved heart health and reduced need for medications. Over a 12-month period, his cholesterol levels normalised, his CRP levels decreased, and his need for antihypertensive medications was eliminated.

Another case involved a 65-year-old female with a history of multiple stents and persistent chest pain. After enrolling in a structured lifestyle program that emphasised dietary changes, daily exercise, and mindfulness practices, she reported a significant reduction in symptoms and improved quality of life. Her LDL cholesterol decreased by 40% without the use of statins, and her exercise tolerance increased dramatically.

These real-life cases illustrate how lifestyle modifications can lead to meaningful improvements in heart health, reducing dependence on medications and enhancing overall well-being.

Integrating Lifestyle Changes into Clinical Practice

Healthcare Integration

Integrating lifestyle medicine into traditional clinical practice requires collaboration between dietitians, physical therapists, and physicians to provide a holistic approach to CAD management. This model ensures that patients receive comprehensive support and guidance in making sustainable lifestyle changes. Group-based programs, such as those pioneered by Dr. Dean Ornish, provide a structured environment where patients can learn and implement lifestyle modifications under professional supervision.

Advanced Preventive Strategies

Personalised Health Approaches

Advances in genetic screening and lipid profiling allow for tailored prevention strategies that enhance the efficacy of lifestyle interventions based on individual risk factors. For example, patients with genetic predispositions to higher cholesterol levels or inflammatory responses can benefit from targeted dietary modifications, specific exercise regimens, and personalised stress reduction techniques.

The Need for Alternative Approaches: Reinforcing the Science

Despite the widespread use of pharmaceutical therapies, their limitations necessitate a more comprehensive approach to CAD management. Many medications address only the symptoms or biochemical markers of disease rather than its root causes. For instance, while statins lower LDL cholesterol, they do not fully address the underlying inflammatory processes that drive plaque formation and destabilisation.

Emerging research supports the notion that alternative, non-pharmacological approaches can offer comparable or superior benefits. For instance, the PREDIMED (Prevención con Dieta Mediterránea) study found that a Mediterranean diet supplemented with extra-virgin olive oil or nuts reduced the incidence of major cardiovascular events by approximately 30% compared to a low-fat diet (Estruch et al., 2013). Similarly, a study by Ornish et al. (1998) demonstrated that comprehensive lifestyle changes could reverse CAD, with participants showing regression of atherosclerosis as evidenced by angiography.

These findings reinforce the potential of lifestyle interventions to complement or, in some cases, replace pharmaceutical treatments. By addressing the root causes of CAD—such as inflammation, oxidative stress, and endothelial dysfunction—lifestyle modifications can provide long-lasting benefits that extend beyond mere symptom management.

Conclusion

This chapter consolidates the scientific evidence supporting lifestyle modifications as potent interventions for CAD, advocating for a cultural shift in heart disease management that prioritises sustainable lifestyle changes over pharmacological interventions. This holistic approach not only treats CAD but also enhances overall quality of life, empowering patients to take control of their health in a proactive, informed manner. As we move forward, it is essential that healthcare providers and patients alike embrace these strategies, recognising that the path to heart health lies not in a single pill or procedure, but in the daily choices we make that nurture and protect the cardiovascular system.

Summary: Lifestyle Approaches to Managing Coronary Artery Disease

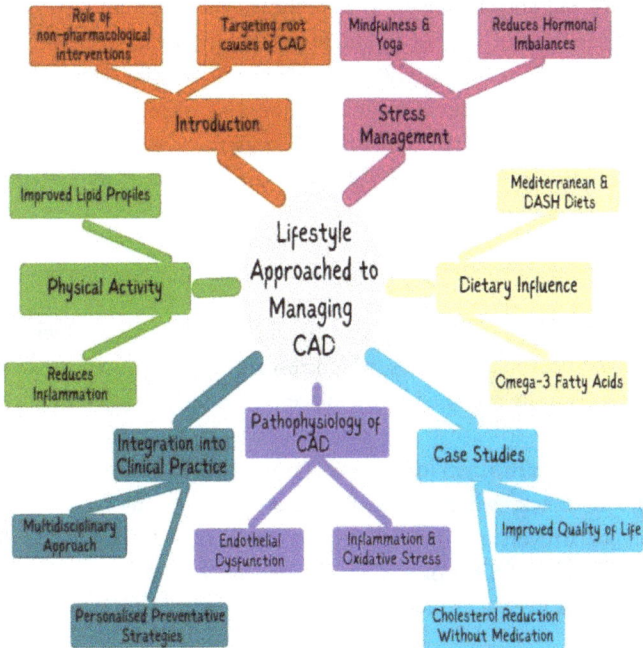

Chapter 4
Angioplasty and Stents: A Critical Look

Introduction

Angioplasty and stenting have become some of the most common procedures for managing coronary artery disease (CAD), particularly for patients presenting with symptoms like chest pain (angina) or those who have experienced a heart attack. These interventions are often seen as definitive solutions, but their widespread use has sparked significant debate within the medical community. While they can be life-saving in acute situations, their necessity and effectiveness in stable CAD have been increasingly called into question. This chapter critically examines the role of angioplasty and stenting, explores their benefits and limitations, and advocates for non-pharmacological and lifestyle approaches supported by emerging scientific evidence.

Understanding Angioplasty and Stents

Angioplasty involves the use of a small balloon to widen blocked or narrowed coronary arteries, which restores blood flow to the heart. This is typically followed by the placement of a stent—a small, wire-mesh tube—to keep the artery open. These procedures are commonly performed in cases of acute coronary syndrome, such as a heart attack, where immediate restoration of blood flow can prevent irreversible damage to the heart muscle. However, the effectiveness of these procedures in managing stable coronary artery disease has been increasingly questioned.

The Controversy: Overuse and Limited Efficacy

Overuse in Stable CAD

Studies have suggested that angioplasty and stenting are frequently overused, particularly in patients with stable CAD who are not experiencing acute symptoms. According to research published in the *New England Journal of Medicine* (Fihn et al., 2012), in many cases, these procedures do not significantly reduce the risk of heart attack or death compared to non-invasive treatments such as lifestyle changes and non-pharmacological therapies. This raises critical questions about whether these invasive interventions should be the first-line treatment for stable CAD, or if other approaches should be prioritised.

Recent Clinical Trials Questioning Efficacy

Recent clinical trials have provided compelling evidence that challenges the traditional role of angioplasty and stenting in stable CAD management:

The ORBITA Trial: The ORBITA trial (Al-Lamee et al., 2018) was a randomised, double-blind, placebo-controlled study that investigated the symptomatic benefit of percutaneous coronary intervention (PCI) in patients with stable angina. Surprisingly, the trial found no significant difference in improvement of symptoms and exercise performance between patients undergoing stenting and those receiving a placebo procedure. This trial has sparked significant debate within the cardiology community and highlighted the need for reevaluation of stenting in the management of chronic stable angina.

The COURAGE Trial: The COURAGE (Clinical Outcomes Utilising Revascularisation and Aggressive Drug Evaluation) trial similarly concluded that initial stent placement for stable CAD offered no additional benefit in preventing heart attacks or death over comprehensive lifestyle interventions. This landmark study demonstrated that lifestyle modifications that include dietary changes, regular exercise, and smoking cessation could provide equivalent or even superior outcomes to invasive procedures in stable CAD patients (Boden et al., 2007).

The Role of Lifestyle Interventions in CAD Management

Lifestyle Interventions: Addressing the Root Causes

Unlike pharmacological approaches that primarily address symptoms or biochemical markers, lifestyle modifications target the root causes of CAD, such as inflammation, oxidative stress, and endothelial dysfunction. By reducing systemic inflammation and improving overall cardiovascular health, lifestyle interventions can significantly reduce the risk of CAD progression. Key lifestyle interventions include:

- **Dietary Modifications:** Diets rich in anti-inflammatory foods, such as the Mediterranean diet, have been shown to reduce systemic inflammation and improve cardiovascular outcomes (Estruch et al., 2013). These diets emphasise the consumption of fruits, vegetables, whole grains, nuts, seeds, and healthy fats like extra-virgin olive oil, all of which contribute to improved heart health.

- **Regular Physical Activity:** Exercise enhances cardiovascular fitness, improves blood pressure, and reduces the risk of CAD progression. Aerobic exercise has been shown to increase endothelial nitric oxide production, which promotes vasodilation and improved vascular health (Hambrecht et al., 2004).

- **Smoking Cessation:** Quitting smoking is one of the most impactful lifestyle changes for reducing cardiovascular risk, as smoking is a major contributor to endothelial dysfunction and atherosclerosis (Bullen, 2008). Smoking cessation reduces the pro-inflammatory state induced by smoking and decreases oxidative stress on the vascular system.

- **Stress Management:** Chronic stress exacerbates CAD by promoting inflammation and increasing blood pressure. Techniques like yoga, meditation, and mindfulness have been shown to reduce stress and improve heart health (Lavretsky et al., 2013). These interventions can decrease the levels of stress hormones like cortisol, which are linked to inflammation and cardiovascular risk.

These lifestyle interventions not only reduce the risk of CAD but also offer numerous additional health benefits, such as improved metabolic function, better mental health, and enhanced quality of life.

Scientific Support for Lifestyle-Based Interventions

Scientific evidence strongly supports the role of lifestyle interventions in preventing and managing CAD. The Lyon Diet Heart Study (de Lorgeril et al., 1999) found that patients who adhered to a Mediterranean-style diet experienced a 70% reduction in all-cause mortality and a 73% reduction in cardiovascular mortality compared to those following a standard low-fat diet. Similarly, the PREDIMED (Prevención con Dieta Mediterránea) study demonstrated that a Mediterranean diet supplemented with extra-virgin olive oil or nuts reduced the incidence of major cardiovascular events by approximately 30% compared to a low-fat diet (Estruch et al., 2013).

These findings underscore the potential of dietary interventions to complement or even replace invasive treatments in certain populations. By addressing the root causes of CAD—such as chronic inflammation and oxidative stress—dietary modifications can significantly improve cardiovascular health and reduce the need for more aggressive interventions.

Patient Stories and Real-World Outcomes

Real-world experiences often provide powerful testimony to the effectiveness of non-invasive approaches in managing CAD. Consider the story of James, a 58-year-old man diagnosed with stable CAD. James was initially recommended to undergo angioplasty and stenting. However, after researching the potential risks and benefits, he decided to explore non-invasive options. With the guidance of a multidisciplinary team, James adopted a plant-based diet, incorporated daily exercise, and began practising stress reduction techniques like meditation.

Over the course of a year, James experienced significant improvements in his health. His cholesterol levels decreased, his angina symptoms subsided, and his exercise tolerance increased. Most importantly, follow-up imaging showed no progression of his arterial plaques. James's experience illustrates that, with the right support and commitment, non-invasive approaches can lead to the successful management of CAD without the need for invasive procedures.

Economic and Psychological Implications of Angioplasty and Stenting

Cost-Effectiveness of Non-Invasive Approaches

The economic impact of the widespread use of angioplasty and stenting, especially in cases where they may not be necessary, is significant. The cost of these procedures can be prohibitive, particularly when considering that non-invasive treatments like lifestyle interventions can provide similar outcomes at a substantially lower cost. Studies assessing cost-effectiveness, such as those found in the *American Heart Journal* (Cohen et al., 2011), often reveal that non-invasive treatments not only offer comparable clinical benefits but also reduce healthcare costs by avoiding unnecessary procedures and hospitalisations.

Patient Preferences and Quality of Life

The psychological impact of undergoing invasive procedures can be profound. Some patients experience increased anxiety and stress due to the invasiveness and potential complications associated with angioplasty and stenting. On the other hand, some individuals feel reassured by such interventions, believing that they offer a definitive solution to their heart disease. Evaluating patient-centred outcomes is crucial for personalised care. A study published in *Circulation* (Sedlis et al., 2009) found that patients managed with lifestyle modifications reported similar or better quality of life outcomes compared to those undergoing stenting, particularly when their expectations were aligned with the treatment strategy.

Beyond Angioplasty: The Case for Non-Pharmacological and Non-Conventional Approaches

With mounting evidence questioning the necessity of angioplasty and stenting in stable CAD, it is imperative to consider alternative strategies that prioritise patient well-being and address the root causes of cardiovascular disease. Non-pharmacological and non-conventional approaches offer a compelling alternative that can be tailored to the individual's needs and preferences.

Anti-Inflammatory and Nutritional Therapies

Anti-inflammatory therapies, including the use of supplements like omega-3 fatty acids, Coenzyme Q10, and magnesium, have shown promise in reducing cardiovascular risk. The PREDIMED study (Estruch et al., 2013) demonstrated that a Mediterranean diet supplemented with extra-virgin olive oil or nuts significantly reduced cardiovascular events. Nutritional interventions that emphasise anti-inflammatory and endothelial-protective nutrients can modulate key pathways involved in CAD.

Mind-Body Therapies

Mind-body therapies such as yoga, meditation, and Tai Chi have been shown to reduce stress, lower blood pressure, and improve endothelial function. A meta-analysis published in *Frontiers in Cardiovascular Medicine* (Lavretsky et al., 2013) found that mind-body practices were associated with improved cardiovascular outcomes and reduced inflammatory markers. These therapies are particularly beneficial for patients with high levels of stress or anxiety, which are known contributors to CAD progression.

Regenerative and Complementary Approaches

Emerging regenerative therapies, such as stem cell treatment and platelet-rich plasma (PRP) therapy, hold potential for repairing damaged cardiac tissue and improving heart function. While these therapies are still in the experimental stage, preliminary studies suggest that they may offer new avenues for non-invasive management of CAD in the future (Vagnozzi et al., 2020).

Conclusion

The current scientific evidence and patient experiences call for a more judicious use of angioplasty and stents, particularly in stable CAD patients. Emphasising lifestyle interventions and non-conventional approaches as first-line treatments could lead to better health outcomes, reduced healthcare costs, and improved patient satisfaction. As research continues to evolve, it is crucial for healthcare providers and patients to engage in shared decision-making that considers not only the clinical benefits of each intervention but also the individual's values, preferences, and overall quality of life. By embracing a broader, more integrative approach to CAD management, we can empower patients to take control of their heart health in ways that extend beyond the limits of traditional medicine.

Summary: Angioplasty and Stents: A Critical Look

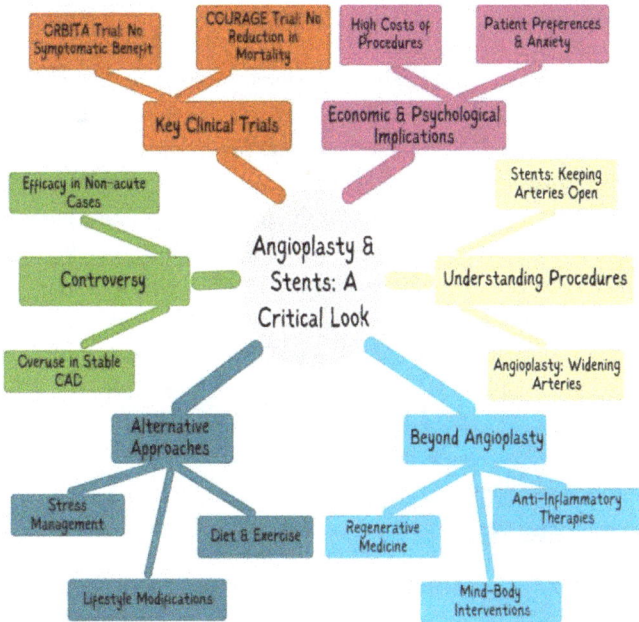

Chapter 5
Lifestyle-Based Therapy vs. Interventional Procedures: A Critical Analysis

Introduction

The management of heart conditions often presents a choice between lifestyle-based approaches and interventional surgical procedures. For decades, interventional procedures like angioplasty and stent placement have been the cornerstone of treating coronary artery disease (CAD), particularly in emergency settings. However, as our understanding of heart disease evolves, it is becoming increasingly evident that lifestyle-based therapy, which encompasses dietary changes, exercise, stress management, and other non-pharmacological strategies, can be equally—if not more—effective in managing stable CAD and preventing cardiovascular events. This chapter delves into the effectiveness and outcomes of these options, presenting research findings and case studies that favour a non-invasive approach and highlight the benefits of lifestyle-based interventions over invasive procedures.

The Case for Lifestyle-Based Therapy

Lifestyle-based therapy involves a combination of dietary modifications, physical activity, stress management, and regular monitoring to target the underlying causes of heart disease, such as hypertension, high cholesterol, obesity, and chronic inflammation. Unlike interventional procedures that address the symptoms or anatomical issues of CAD, lifestyle interventions can influence the systemic processes that lead to the development and progression of heart disease. By targeting these root causes, lifestyle-based therapy offers a holistic approach that not only manages symptoms but also improves overall cardiovascular health.

Scientific Backing for Lifestyle-Based Interventions

Research consistently shows that for many patients, particularly those with stable CAD, lifestyle-based therapy can be as effective as surgical interventions in preventing major cardiovascular events. Studies like the COURAGE trial and the Lifestyle Heart Trial have demonstrated that non-invasive strategies can lead to outcomes comparable to those achieved with stenting and surgery.

The COURAGE Trial: This landmark study (Boden et al., 2007) compared outcomes in patients with stable CAD who were managed with lifestyle-based therapy alone versus those who underwent initial stenting and lifestyle changes. The results showed no significant difference in the risk of heart attack, need for urgent revascularisation, or death from coronary artery disease between the two groups over a five-year period. These findings challenge the traditional view that interventional procedures are superior for managing stable CAD.

The Lifestyle Heart Trial: This groundbreaking study by Dr. Dean Ornish (1990) demonstrated that comprehensive lifestyle changes, including a low-fat vegetarian diet, regular exercise, stress management, and social support, could not only stabilise but also reverse coronary artery disease. Participants who adhered to the lifestyle intervention showed regression of atherosclerosis as evidenced by angiography, along with significant reductions in angina symptoms and improved quality of life.

Benefits Beyond Symptom Management

Lifestyle-based therapy offers benefits that extend beyond the management of heart disease symptoms. These interventions reduce the risk of comorbid conditions such as type 2 diabetes, hypertension, and obesity. For example, a plant-based diet rich in anti-inflammatory foods can lower blood pressure, improve cholesterol levels, and reduce systemic inflammation. Regular physical activity enhances endothelial function, increases insulin sensitivity, and promotes weight loss. Stress management techniques like yoga and meditation can lower cortisol levels, reduce blood pressure, and improve heart rate variability, all of which contribute to better cardiovascular health.

Interventional Procedures: Immediate Relief vs. Long-Term Benefit

Common interventional procedures for CAD include angioplasty and stenting, which are often recommended for acute cases, such as myocardial infarction, or where there is significant arterial blockage. While these procedures can provide immediate relief from symptoms and are life-saving in emergency situations, their benefits in stable patients over the long term are less definitive.

Immediate Relief: The Primary Advantage

In acute settings, such as during a heart attack, restoring blood flow to the heart muscle as quickly as possible is critical to prevent irreversible damage. In these scenarios, angioplasty and stenting can be life-saving and are the preferred treatment options. However, when it comes to stable CAD, where the goal is to prevent disease progression and reduce the risk of future events, lifestyle-based therapy offers a sustainable approach that addresses the disease's root causes.

The Limitations of Interventional Procedures

Interventional procedures can sometimes mask the underlying systemic processes that contribute to heart disease, such as chronic inflammation and endothelial dysfunction. A patient may experience symptom relief following a stent placement, but without addressing the underlying issues, the disease process continues. This can lead to recurrent symptoms, progression of atherosclerosis in other arteries, and the need for additional interventions.

Studies have shown that in patients with stable CAD, stenting does not significantly reduce the risk of heart attack or death compared to lifestyle-based approaches. The FAME 2 trial (2012) found that while stenting reduced the need for urgent revascularisation, it did not improve the overall risk of heart attack or death in stable CAD patients when compared to lifestyle-based therapy.

Comparative Effectiveness: Research Findings

A review of several studies published in the *New England Journal of Medicine* (2017) compared the long-term effectiveness of stents versus lifestyle-based treatments and found no significant difference in the risk of heart attack, need for urgent revascularisation, or death from coronary artery disease. This evidence suggests that for stable CAD patients, lifestyle interventions should be considered as the first-line approach.

Case Studies: Lifestyle-Based Therapy in Action

Case Study 1: John's Story

John, a 58-year-old man with stable angina, was initially recommended to undergo angioplasty and stenting. After discussing his options with his cardiologist and doing his own research, he decided to try lifestyle-based therapy first. Over the course of a year, John adopted a plant-based diet, began exercising regularly, and incorporated stress management techniques like yoga and mindfulness meditation into his daily routine. Not only did his angina symptoms improve, but follow-up tests also showed no progression in his CAD. His cholesterol levels dropped, his blood pressure normalised, and he felt more energetic and engaged in life.

Case Study 2: Sarah's Journey

Sarah, a 62-year-old woman with a history of chronic chest pain, underwent stenting for her CAD. While the procedure was initially successful, she experienced re-narrowing of her arteries (restenosis) within a year, leading to additional interventions. Frustrated by the recurrent procedures, Sarah turned to lifestyle-based therapy. She began a Mediterranean diet, engaged in regular physical activity, and practised mindfulness meditation. Over time, her symptoms improved, and she was able to discontinue several of her medications. Sarah's experience highlights the potential for lifestyle interventions to provide long-term stability and quality of life improvements without the need for repeated procedures.

Analogueies to Explain Concepts

Analogueies can simplify complex concepts and help patients understand the differences between lifestyle-based therapy and interventional procedures:

- **The Garden Hose Analoguey:** If a garden hose is clogged, squeezing it (angioplasty) or inserting a support (stent) might immediately improve water flow. However, cleaning it out and regularly maintaining it (lifestyle-based therapy) prevents clogs from occurring in the first place, providing a more sustainable solution.

- **The Band-Aid vs. Healing Salve Analoguey:** While a Band-Aid (stent) might cover up a wound and provide a temporary fix, a healing salve (lifestyle-based therapy) treats the underlying conditions that caused the wound, promoting long-term healing.

These analogueies emphasise that while interventional procedures can provide temporary relief, lifestyle-based therapy addresses the root causes of CAD and offers sustainable, long-term benefits.

Economic and Quality of Life Considerations

Economic Benefits of Lifestyle-Based Therapy

Lifestyle-based therapy not only tends to be more cost-effective than interventional procedures but also reduces the risk of complications associated with surgery. A study published in the *Journal of the American College of Cardiology* (2018) found that lifestyle interventions led to a significant reduction in healthcare costs due to decreased hospital admissions, fewer medications, and lower rates of recurrent procedures. These savings can be substantial, particularly for patients with chronic conditions like CAD.

Quality of Life Improvements

Patients who adopt lifestyle-based therapy often report a higher quality of life compared to those who undergo interventional procedures. They experience improvements in energy levels, mental clarity, and overall well-being. Engaging in lifestyle changes also fosters a sense of empowerment, as patients feel more in control of their health and are actively contributing to their own recovery. This psychological benefit can enhance adherence to treatment and lead to better long-term outcomes.

Conclusion

The evidence and case studies presented in this chapter suggest that while interventional procedures are crucial in acute settings, lifestyle-based therapy offers a viable, effective alternative for managing chronic heart conditions. By emphasising dietary modifications, physical activity, stress management, and other non-pharmacological strategies, patients can achieve substantial improvements in cardiac health without the need for invasive procedures. As healthcare moves towards a more patient-centred approach, lifestyle-based therapy should be prioritised as the first-line treatment for stable CAD, offering a holistic, sustainable path to long-term heart health and well-being.

Summary:Lifestyle-Based Therapy vs. Interventional Procedures: A Critical Analysis

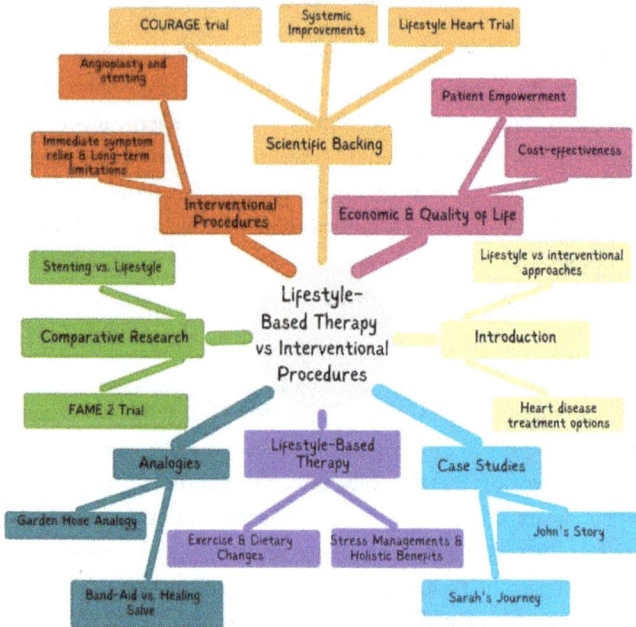

Chapter 6
The Impact of Diet and Lifestyle on Heart Health

Introduction

The profound influence of diet and lifestyle on cardiovascular health cannot be overstated. Cardiovascular diseases (CVD) remain the leading cause of mortality globally, but emerging research underscores that many of these conditions are preventable through non-pharmacological means. By making specific dietary choices, engaging in regular physical activity, and employing stress management techniques, individuals can significantly enhance their heart health and reduce the risk of disease. This chapter explores how these lifestyle interventions not only contribute to cardiovascular well-being but also interact with other body systems to promote whole-body health, supported by scientific evidence, clinical studies, and insights from leading cardiologists such as Dr Aseem Malhotra.

Dietary Influences on Heart Health

Heart-Healthy Diets: A Nutritional Foundation for Cardiovascular Health

Nutrition plays a pivotal role in modulating cardiovascular risk factors. Diets rich in anti-inflammatory and cardioprotective nutrients have been shown to improve cholesterol levels, reduce systemic inflammation, and support healthy blood pressure. Two of the most well-researched diets for heart health include the Mediterranean and DASH (Dietary Approaches to Stop Hypertension) diets. Additionally, new perspectives like Dr Aseem Malhotra's Pioppi Diet have gained recognition for their comprehensive, science-backed approach to heart health.

Mediterranean Diet: Characterised by high consumption of olive oil, fruits, vegetables, whole grains, nuts, and fish, the Mediterranean diet has long been associated with a lower risk of cardiovascular diseases. The landmark PREDIMED study (Estruch et al., 2013) published in the *New England Journal of Medicine* demonstrated that individuals following this diet experienced a significant reduction in the incidence of major cardiovascular events, including heart attack and stroke. The study found that participants who supplemented their diet with extra-virgin olive oil or nuts had a 30% lower risk of cardiovascular events compared to those on a low-fat diet. The Mediterranean diet's high content of monounsaturated fats and polyphenols helps reduce oxidative stress, a key contributor to atherosclerosis.

The Pioppi Diet: Developed by Dr Aseem Malhotra, the Pioppi Diet takes inspiration from the lifestyles of the residents of Pioppi, a small village in Southern Italy renowned for its residents' exceptional longevity and low rates of heart disease. The diet emphasises natural, whole foods with a focus on healthy fats, fibrous vegetables, and minimal processed carbohydrates. Dr Malhotra advocates for the consumption of high-quality fats, such as those found in extra-virgin olive oil, nuts, and fatty fish, which have been shown to support cardiovascular health. His research, published in the *British Journal of Sports Medicine* (Malhotra et al., 2017), challenges the traditional view of saturated fats and heart disease, suggesting that inflammation, rather than cholesterol levels alone, plays a critical role in cardiovascular risk. The Pioppi Diet, therefore, prioritises reducing systemic inflammation through dietary and lifestyle modifications rather than focusing solely on cholesterol reduction.

Dr Malhotra's work has helped shift the paradigm in cardiovascular nutrition by emphasising the importance of lifestyle factors such as stress management, sleep, and intermittent fasting, all of which are integral components of the Pioppi Diet. His approach aligns with the growing body of evidence that underscores the significance of a comprehensive lifestyle strategy in reducing cardiovascular risk.

DASH Diet: Explicitly developed to combat high blood pressure, the DASH diet emphasises fruits, vegetables, whole grains, lean proteins, and low-fat dairy while minimising sodium, refined sugars, and saturated fats. Research published in *Hypertension* (Appel et al., 1997) revealed that the DASH diet significantly lowers systolic and diastolic blood pressure, reducing the risk of hypertension—a major risk factor for heart disease. The diet's emphasis on potassium, magnesium, and calcium promotes vasodilation and endothelial function, contributing to its heart-protective effects.

Components of a Heart-Healthy Diet: Beyond the Basics

Certain foods and nutrients have been identified as particularly beneficial for cardiovascular health due to their ability to modulate inflammation, improve lipid profiles, and support endothelial function.

- **Omega-3 Fatty Acids:** Found abundantly in fatty fish like salmon, sardines, and mackerel, as well as in plant-based sources like flaxseeds and chia seeds, omega-3s are known for their anti-inflammatory properties. A meta-analysis published in *Circulation* (Mozaffarian & Rimm, 2006) found that regular consumption of omega-3-rich foods reduced the risk of fatal heart attacks by 35%. Omega-3s decrease triglyceride levels, lower blood pressure, and prevent arrhythmias, making them a cornerstone of a heart-healthy diet.
- **Fibre-Rich Foods:** Dietary fibre, particularly soluble fibre found in oats, fruits, and vegetables, helps reduce LDL cholesterol by binding bile acids in the gut and promoting their excretion. The *Journal of Nutrition* (2005) reported that individuals consuming a diet high in soluble fibre had a 7% reduction in LDL cholesterol, which directly translates to a lower risk of heart disease.

- **Plant Sterols and Stanols:** These compounds, naturally present in small amounts in foods like vegetable oils, nuts, and seeds, help block the absorption of cholesterol in the intestines. Adding plant sterols and stanols to the diet can lower LDL cholesterol by 5-15%, according to research published in *Atherosclerosis* (2003). This reduction is significant enough to warrant the inclusion of these compounds in dietary guidelines for heart health.

- **Anti-Inflammatory Foods:** Dr Malhotra's Pioppi Diet emphasises the inclusion of anti-inflammatory foods such as leafy greens, berries, and cruciferous vegetables. These foods are rich in antioxidants like polyphenols and flavonoids, which neutralise free radicals and reduce inflammation, a key driver of cardiovascular disease. Dr Malhotra's research highlights that addressing inflammation through diet can have a greater impact on heart health than cholesterol management alone.

Physical Activity and Heart Health

Role of Exercise in Cardiovascular Fitness: More Than Just Cardio

Exercise is a powerful tool for improving cardiovascular health and overall physical well-being. Regular physical activity strengthens the heart muscle, enhances endothelial function, and promotes better circulation. Different types of exercise contribute uniquely to heart health:

- **Aerobic Exercise:** Activities like walking, running, and cycling are well-known for their cardiovascular benefits. Aerobic exercise improves oxygen utilisation, enhances cardiac output, and reduces blood pressure. A meta-analysis in *Circulation* (2016) found that individuals who engage in regular aerobic exercise have a 20-35% lower risk of cardiovascular disease and related mortality compared to those who are inactive.

- **Resistance Training:** Incorporating moderate resistance training helps maintain muscle mass, improves metabolism, and supports heart health. A study in the *American Journal of Medicine*

(2012) found that resistance training reduced the risk of cardiovascular disease by improving glucose metabolism and reducing visceral fat, which is strongly associated with heart disease.

- **Flexibility and Balance Exercises:** Activities like yoga, Tai Chi, and Pilates not only improve flexibility and balance but also enhance cardiovascular health by promoting relaxation and reducing stress. These exercises support parasympathetic nervous system activation, which lowers heart rate and blood pressure.

Clinical Evidence for Exercise in Heart Disease Prevention

Exercise is one of the most well-supported interventions for preventing and managing heart disease. The Harvard Alumni Study (Paffenbarger et al., 1986) found that men who engaged in regular moderate to vigorous physical activity had a 23% lower risk of heart disease mortality compared to sedentary individuals. Furthermore, a study in the *Journal of the American Heart Association* (2015) concluded that both aerobic and resistance training independently reduced cardiovascular risk, with the greatest benefits observed when the two were combined.

Stress Management and Heart Health

The Impact of Chronic Stress on Cardiovascular Health

Chronic stress is a significant contributor to cardiovascular disease, as it triggers the release of stress hormones like cortisol and adrenaline, which increase heart rate, blood pressure, and inflammation. Prolonged exposure to these hormones can lead to hypertension, arterial damage, and increased risk of atherosclerosis. Addressing chronic stress is, therefore, a critical component of heart health.

Effective Stress Management Techniques

Various stress management techniques have been shown to lower blood pressure, reduce heart rate, and improve overall heart health. Some of the most effective methods include:

- **Mindfulness and Meditation:** Practices such as mindfulness-based stress reduction (MBSR) and meditation have been shown to lower blood pressure and heart rate, reducing the risk of heart disease. A study published in *Hypertension* (2013) found that participants who practised transcendental meditation for 20 minutes twice daily had a 48% lower risk of heart attack and stroke compared to those who did not meditate.

- **Yoga and Raj Yoga:** Yoga combines physical postures, breathing exercises, and meditation to reduce stress and improve cardiovascular health. Studies in journals like *The Lancet* have documented its benefits in improving cardiac efficiency, enhancing endothelial function, and reducing stress markers. Raj Yoga, a form of meditative practice that emphasises mental relaxation and emotional resilience, has been shown to lower blood pressure and reduce stress-induced arrhythmias.

Integrating Stress Management with Heart Health

Integrating stress management techniques into heart health strategies can create a synergistic effect, enhancing the benefits of diet and exercise. For example, combining regular yoga practice with a heart-healthy diet can lead to greater reductions in blood pressure and improvements in arterial health than either intervention alone. A holistic approach that includes stress management addresses the psychological and emotional factors that contribute to cardiovascular disease, offering a comprehensive strategy for heart health.

The Whole-Body Impact of Lifestyle Interventions:
Beyond the Heart

Emerging evidence suggests that lifestyle interventions not only benefit the cardiovascular system but also have profound effects on other body systems, creating a ripple effect that enhances overall health and well-being. This interconnectedness is due to the complex interplay between cardiovascular health and other physiological processes, such as immune function, hormonal balance, and metabolic health.

The Gut-Heart Axis: Linking Nutrition and Cardiovascular Health

The gut microbiome plays a crucial role in modulating inflammation, cholesterol metabolism, and blood pressure regulation. Diets rich in fibre, polyphenols, and fermented foods support a healthy gut microbiome, which in turn contributes to cardiovascular health. A study published in *Nature Medicine* (2019) found that individuals with a diverse and balanced gut microbiome had lower levels of trimethylamine N-oxide (TMAO), a compound linked to an increased risk of heart disease.

The Role of Hormones in Cardiovascular Health

Hormonal imbalances, such as those seen in menopause or in conditions like hypothyroidism, can significantly impact heart health. Lifestyle interventions that promote hormonal balance—such as stress management, regular physical activity, and a nutrient-rich diet—can help mitigate these effects. For example, phytooestrogens found in foods like soy can help balance oestrogen levels in postmenopausal women, reducing their risk of heart disease.

The Brain-Heart Connection: Mental Health and Cardiovascular Risk

There is a bidirectional relationship between mental health and heart health. Depression, anxiety, and chronic stress are all associated with increased cardiovascular risk, while heart disease can exacerbate mental health conditions. Integrating mental health support, such as therapy or mindfulness practices, into heart health strategies can reduce the risk of cardiovascular events and improve overall quality of life.

Case Studies: Real-World Success with Lifestyle Interventions

John's Transformation: A Diet and Exercise Success Story

John, a 55-year-old man with a history of high blood pressure and high cholesterol, was initially advised to start statins and antihypertensives. However, he chose to focus on lifestyle changes instead. After six months of adopting a Mediterranean and Pioppi-inspired diet, engaging in daily aerobic exercise, and practising mindfulness meditation, John's blood pressure normalised, his cholesterol levels improved, and his inflammatory markers decreased. His doctor noted that John's cardiovascular risk had significantly reduced, and he no longer needed medication.

Sarah's Journey: The Power of Integrating Diet and Stress Management

Sarah, a 62-year-old woman with stable angina, experienced recurrent chest pain despite multiple stent placements. Frustrated with her limited progress, she began a comprehensive lifestyle program that included a plant-based diet, regular yoga, and stress management through mindfulness. Within a year, Sarah reported a dramatic reduction in chest pain, improved exercise tolerance, and an enhanced sense of well-being. Her cardiologist noted that Sarah's condition had stabilised, and no further interventions were required.

Integrating Diet, Exercise, and Stress Management: A Holistic Approach to Heart Health

Combining dietary improvements, regular physical activity, and effective stress management creates a synergistic effect that greatly enhances heart health. This holistic approach is supported by numerous studies demonstrating its superior benefits over any single intervention alone. For example, the Ornish Lifestyle Medicine

Program, which integrates all three components, has been shown to not only stabilise but also reverse coronary artery disease in a majority of patients (Ornish et al., 1998).

Conclusion

This chapter underscores the critical importance of diet, exercise, and stress management in maintaining and enhancing cardiovascular health. By adopting a comprehensive lifestyle approach, individuals can significantly improve their heart health outcomes and reduce the need for pharmacological interventions. This integrated strategy not only supports cardiovascular function but also enhances overall well-being and quality of life, empowering individuals to take proactive steps toward their health. As research continues to unveil the interconnectedness of body systems, it becomes clear that addressing heart health through lifestyle interventions is not only effective but also essential for holistic health and longevity.

Summary: The Impact of Diet and Lifestyle on Heart Health

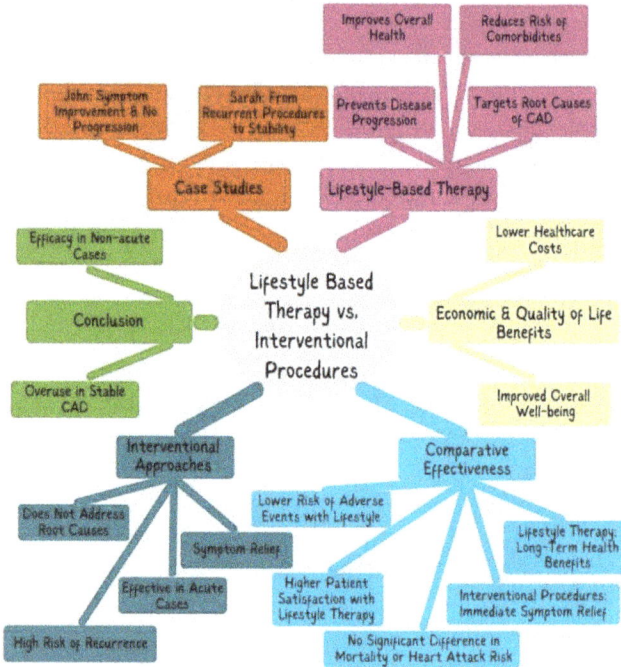

Chapter 7
The Value of Breathwork in Coronary Artery Disease (CAD)

Breathwork, the conscious regulation of breathing patterns, has emerged as a powerful tool for managing various health conditions, including coronary artery disease (CAD). While traditionally considered a component of yoga and meditation, breathwork has gained recognition as a standalone therapeutic practice supported by scientific evidence. It offers a non-pharmacological, non-invasive intervention that can enhance cardiovascular health by modulating physiological processes such as heart rate, blood pressure, and autonomic nervous system balance. This chapter explores the value of breathwork in CAD, supported by scientific research, clinical applications, and various types of breathwork practices.

Understanding Coronary Artery Disease and the Role of Breathwork

Coronary artery disease, characterised by the narrowing or blockage of coronary arteries due to the build-up of atherosclerotic plaques, is a leading cause of morbidity and mortality worldwide. The pathophysiology of CAD involves complex interactions between cholesterol deposition, inflammation, oxidative stress, and endothelial dysfunction. Traditional management strategies focus on medications and lifestyle modifications such as diet and exercise. However, breathwork provides an additional, often overlooked modality that targets key physiological processes contributing to CAD.

Breathwork influences cardiovascular health through multiple mechanisms:

1. **Modulating the Autonomic Nervous System (ANS):** Breathwork practices such as slow, deep breathing activate the parasympathetic nervous system (rest-and-digest response), promoting relaxation, reducing heart rate, and lowering blood pressure. This modulation is critical in patients with CAD, as chronic sympathetic overactivity (fight-or-flight response) is linked to increased cardiovascular risk.

2. **Reducing Inflammation and Oxidative Stress:** Breathwork techniques like diaphragmatic breathing and alternate nostril breathing have been shown to decrease markers of inflammation and oxidative stress, which are key contributors to CAD progression.

3. **Improving Heart Rate Variability (HRV):** HRV, a measure of the variation in time between consecutive heartbeats, reflects the balance between the sympathetic and parasympathetic branches of the ANS. Higher HRV is associated with better cardiovascular health and reduced risk of arrhythmias and sudden cardiac events. Breathwork practices enhance HRV, making them beneficial for CAD management.

4. **Lowering Blood Pressure:** Hypertension is a major risk factor for CAD. Breathwork, especially techniques like slow breathing, has been shown to lower blood pressure by enhancing baroreflex sensitivity and promoting vasodilation.

5. **Improving Oxygen Utilisation and Tissue Perfusion:** Certain breathwork practices, such as the Buteyko method, optimise oxygen delivery and utilisation at the cellular level, improving overall cardiovascular efficiency.

Scientific Evidence Supporting Breathwork in CAD

Numerous studies have explored the effects of breathwork on cardiovascular health, with promising results:

- **Impact on Blood Pressure:** A study published in *Hypertension Research* (2010) investigated the effects of slow, deep breathing (six breaths per minute) on blood pressure and heart rate in patients with hypertension and CAD. The study found significant reductions in both systolic and diastolic blood pressure, along with a decrease in heart rate. The authors attributed these benefits to enhanced parasympathetic activity and improved baroreceptor sensitivity.

- **Heart Rate Variability and Autonomic Function:** Research published in *Frontiers in Physiology* (2017) examined the impact of diaphragmatic breathing on HRV and autonomic balance in CAD patients. The study found that regular practice of diaphragmatic breathing increased HRV and shifted the autonomic balance toward parasympathetic dominance, indicating reduced cardiovascular stress and improved resilience to adverse cardiac events.

- **Reduction in Stress and Inflammatory Markers:** A study in *Psychoneuroendocrinology* (2015) assessed the effects of alternate nostril breathing on cortisol levels and inflammatory markers in individuals with high cardiovascular risk. The results showed a significant decrease in cortisol and C-reactive protein (CRP), suggesting that breathwork can attenuate the stress response and reduce systemic inflammation.

Types of Breathwork for CAD: Techniques and Benefits

There are various breathwork techniques, each with distinct physiological effects and therapeutic benefits. Incorporating these practices into CAD management can provide a holistic approach to cardiovascular health.

1. Diaphragmatic Breathing (Abdominal Breathing)

    a. **Technique:** Diaphragmatic breathing involves engaging the diaphragm during inhalation, allowing the abdomen to expand while keeping the chest relatively still. This technique maximises lung capacity and enhances oxygen exchange.

b. **Benefits for CAD:** Diaphragmatic breathing activates the parasympathetic nervous system, reducing heart rate and blood pressure. It also increases HRV and reduces cortisol levels, promoting a state of relaxation. Regular practice can alleviate symptoms of angina and reduce anxiety associated with CAD.

c. **Scientific Evidence:** A study in the *Journal of Cardiopulmonary Rehabilitation and Prevention* (2018) found that CAD patients who practised diaphragmatic breathing for eight weeks showed significant improvements in HRV, reduced angina frequency, and better exercise tolerance compared to the control group.

2. Slow Breathing (Resonance Breathing)

a. **Technique:** Slow breathing involves reducing the breathing rate to approximately six breaths per minute. This technique is often practised with a focus on smooth and prolonged exhalation.

b. **Benefits for CAD:** Slow breathing enhances baroreflex sensitivity, which is responsible for maintaining blood pressure stability. It also increases parasympathetic activity and improves HRV. Patients with CAD can experience reductions in blood pressure, heart rate, and perceived stress.

c. **Scientific Evidence:** A meta-analysis published in *Current Cardiology Reviews* (2017) concluded that slow breathing techniques significantly reduce blood pressure and heart rate in patients with hypertension and CAD, making it an effective adjunct to conventional therapies.

3. Alternate Nostril Breathing (Nadi Shodhana)

a. **Technique:** This yoga-based technique involves alternating the inhalation and exhalation between the left and right nostrils. It is believed to balance the two hemispheres of the brain and promote autonomic regulation.

b.   **Benefits for CAD:** Alternate nostril breathing reduces sympathetic overactivity, balances the autonomic nervous system, and lowers stress-related hormones. It is particularly beneficial for managing anxiety and emotional stress, which are common in CAD patients.

c.   **Scientific Evidence:** A study in *International Journal of Yoga* (2013) demonstrated that alternate nostril breathing improved HRV and reduced sympathetic dominance in participants, suggesting enhanced cardiovascular resilience and reduced stress reactivity.

4.   **Buteyko Breathing**

a.   **Technique:** The Buteyko method involves shallow, nasal breathing with a focus on reducing breathing volume and increasing carbon dioxide tolerance. It aims to restore normal breathing patterns and improve oxygen utilisation.

b.   **Benefits for CAD:** Buteyko breathing enhances oxygen delivery to tissues, improves exercise tolerance, and reduces symptoms of dyspnea (shortness of breath) in CAD patients. It also helps control blood pressure and stabilise heart rate.

c.   **Scientific Evidence:** A randomised controlled trial published in *Respiratory Medicine* (2015) found that CAD patients practising Buteyko breathing experienced significant improvements in exercise tolerance and oxygen saturation, along with reductions in dyspnea and fatigue.

5.   **Box Breathing (Square Breathing)**

a.   **Technique:** Box breathing involves inhaling, holding the breath, exhaling, and holding again, each for an equal count (e.g., four counts each). It is often used by athletes and individuals in high-stress professions to maintain calm and focus.

b. **Benefits for CAD:** Box breathing reduces the sympathetic response, lowers heart rate, and decreases blood pressure. It also enhances mental clarity and reduces anxiety, which can be beneficial for CAD patients experiencing stress or panic attacks.

c. **Scientific Evidence:** Although research specific to CAD is limited, studies on box breathing in stress management have shown that it significantly reduces cortisol levels and increases HRV, suggesting potential cardiovascular benefits.

6. **Ujjayi Breathing (Ocean Breath)**

a. **Technique:** Ujjayi breathing, a pranayama technique used in yoga, involves gently constricting the back of the throat during inhalation and exhalation, creating a soft, ocean-like sound. This technique is often combined with physical postures and meditation.

b. **Benefits for CAD:** Ujjayi breathing reduces blood pressure, promotes relaxation, and improves oxygenation. It can be particularly helpful for managing symptoms of anxiety and panic in CAD patients.

c. **Scientific Evidence:** A study in the *Journal of Clinical Hypertension* (2018) found that participants practising Ujjayi breathing along with yoga had significant reductions in blood pressure and heart rate compared to those practising physical postures alone.

Integrating Breathwork into CAD Management: Practical Applications

Breathwork can be integrated into conventional CAD management in several ways, offering both preventive and therapeutic benefits.

Here are practical applications for incorporating breathwork into a comprehensive CAD treatment plan:

1. **Prevention and Risk Reduction:** For individuals at risk of developing CAD, breathwork can serve as a preventive strategy by reducing hypertension, managing stress, and improving HRV. Encouraging patients to practise slow or diaphragmatic breathing for 10-15 minutes daily can help reduce overall cardiovascular risk.

2. **Symptom Management:** For patients with stable CAD or those recovering from a cardiac event, breathwork can help alleviate symptoms such as angina, dyspnea, and palpitations. Techniques like diaphragmatic breathing and alternate nostril breathing can be practised during episodes of anxiety or chest discomfort to promote relaxation and symptom relief.

3. **Rehabilitation and Recovery:** Breathwork can be incorporated into cardiac rehabilitation programs to enhance recovery post-myocardial infarction or surgery. It can improve exercise tolerance, reduce anxiety, and support autonomic balance. Patients can be taught to use techniques like Buteyko breathing or Ujjayi breath during physical rehabilitation exercises to optimise cardiovascular performance.

4. **Stress and Emotional Management:** Emotional stress is a common trigger for cardiac events. Teaching CAD patients breathwork techniques such as box breathing or Ujjayi breathing can provide them with tools to manage acute stress, reduce anxiety, and prevent stress-induced cardiac episodes.

Case Studies: Real-World Applications of Breathwork in CAD

- ### Case Study 1: John's Experience with Diaphragmatic Breathing

John, a 60-year-old man with a history of CAD and hypertension, was experiencing frequent episodes of angina. After learning diaphragmatic breathing as part of his cardiac rehabilitation program, he practised it daily for 15 minutes. Within three months, John reported a significant reduction in angina frequency, improved exercise tolerance, and better control over his blood pressure. His cardiologist noted that his HRV had increased, indicating improved autonomic function.

- ### Case Study 2: Sarah's Journey with Alternate Nostril Breathing

Sarah, a 58-year-old woman diagnosed with CAD and anxiety, found it difficult to manage her symptoms despite medication and lifestyle changes. After attending a yoga workshop, she began practising alternate nostril breathing twice daily. Within six weeks, Sarah experienced reduced anxiety, improved sleep, and a sense of calm. Follow-up tests showed reductions in her CRP levels, suggesting a decrease in systemic inflammation.

Conclusion

Breathwork represents a promising, non-pharmacological intervention for managing CAD. By targeting autonomic regulation, reducing stress and inflammation, and enhancing cardiovascular efficiency, breathwork offers a unique approach that complements traditional medical therapies. With scientific evidence supporting its efficacy, breathwork can be integrated into CAD management to improve patient outcomes, reduce symptom burden, and enhance overall quality of life. As the understanding of breathwork's physiological impact continues to grow, it holds the potential to become a cornerstone of holistic cardiovascular care.

Summary: The Value of Breathwork in Coronary Artery Disease (CAD)

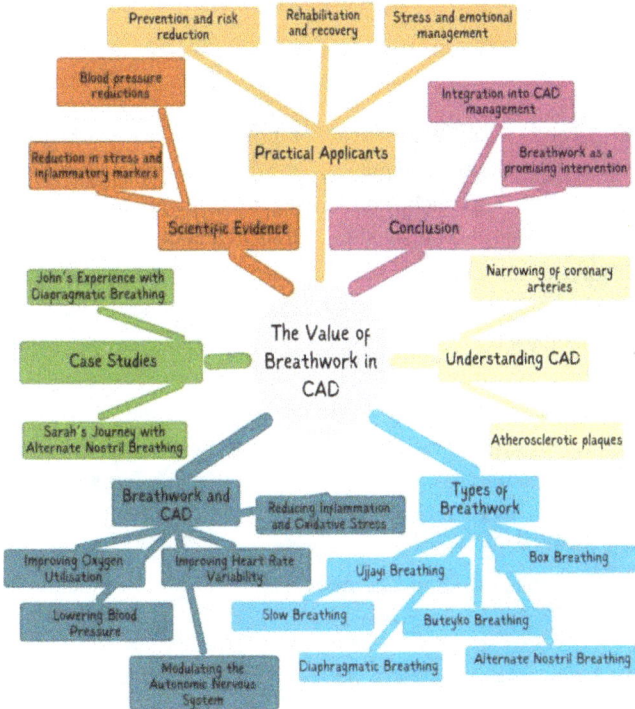

Chapter 8
Patient-Centred Care:
Empowering Choices

Introduction

Patient-centred care is a critical component of modern healthcare, particularly in the management of chronic conditions such as heart disease. This approach emphasises the importance of patient education and choice, enabling individuals to make informed decisions about their treatment options. In the realm of cardiology, where the conventional model often relies heavily on pharmacological interventions, a patient-centred approach offers an alternative that prioritises the patient's values, preferences, and understanding of their health journey. This chapter explores the tools and strategies that facilitate this empowerment, ensuring that patients are active participants in their healthcare. It also highlights the perspectives of thought leaders like Dr. Aseem Malhotra, who advocate for transparency and shared decision-making, particularly regarding the risks and benefits of statin therapy and other pharmacological interventions.

The Importance of Patient Education in Heart Health

Understanding Heart Health: A Foundation for Empowerment

Education is foundational in patient-centred care. Well-informed patients are better equipped to manage their conditions and make decisions that align with their health goals and lifestyle preferences. For heart health, this includes understanding the risk factors, the role of diet and exercise, the impact of stress, and the specifics of any prescribed treatments or procedures. However, the complexity of cardiovascular disease often necessitates that information be tailored to the patient's level of health literacy to ensure comprehension and application.

Studies have shown that patient education can significantly improve health outcomes in cardiovascular care. A systematic review published in the *Journal of Cardiovascular Nursing* (2016) demonstrated that educational interventions led to improved adherence to medication, better lifestyle choices, and reduced hospitalisation rates among heart disease patients. This underscores the importance of structured educational programs in fostering an environment where patients can take charge of their health.

Resources for Education: Bridging Knowledge Gaps

Healthcare facilities such as hospitals and clinics often provide resources like brochures, websites, and workshops that cover various aspects of cardiovascular health. These resources should explain complex medical information in understandable terms, covering topics from the mechanics of heart function to the details of medication regimens. Personalised education, where patients receive information based on their unique health profile, has been shown to be more effective than generic information.

For example, in a study published in *Heart & Lung* (2015), patients who received Personalised education about heart disease risk factors and management strategies demonstrated a higher level of engagement and motivation to adopt lifestyle changes compared to those who received standard educational materials. Personalised educational tools, such as interactive digital platforms and tailored printouts, allow patients to visualise their health metrics and the impact of various lifestyle choices on their cardiovascular risk.

Enhancing Patient Autonomy through Shared Decision-Making

The Concept of Shared Decision-Making

Shared decision-making is a collaborative process in which patients and healthcare providers make health decisions together. This process combines the medical professional's expert knowledge with the patient's values, preferences, and personal experiences. It is particularly relevant in the management of chronic conditions like heart disease, where treatment options can vary significantly in terms of risk, benefit, and alignment with a patient's lifestyle.

Tools like decision aids can be particularly useful in facilitating shared decision-making. These aids provide information about the risks and benefits of each treatment option, presented in an unbiased and accessible manner, and can help patients weigh these in the context of their personal values and lifestyles. Research has shown that the use of decision aids can increase patient knowledge, reduce decisional conflict, and lead to choices that are more consistent with patients' informed preferences.

Dr Aseem Malhotra's Perspective on Informed Consent

Dr Aseem Malhotra, a renowned cardiologist and advocate for evidence-based medicine, has been vocal about the importance of informed consent in cardiovascular treatment, particularly in relation to statins. He argues that many patients are not fully informed about the potential risks and benefits of statin therapy. According to Malhotra, the widespread use of statins has been driven by an overemphasis on cholesterol management without adequate consideration of other factors, such as inflammation and lifestyle.

In his critique published in the *British Medical Journal* (2013), Dr. Malhotra highlights that a significant number of patients may experience side effects such as muscle pain, fatigue, and an increased risk of type 2 diabetes. He calls for greater transparency in discussing these risks and more emphasis on lifestyle interventions, which have been shown to be highly effective in managing cardiovascular risk. This perspective aligns with the patient-centred care model, which prioritises patient autonomy and the right to make fully informed decisions about their health.

Dr Malhotra further advocates for shared decision-making to ensure that patients are provided with a comprehensive view of all available treatment options. He emphasises the need for healthcare providers to present the absolute risk reductions and potential side effects in a transparent manner, allowing patients to weigh the benefits and drawbacks of each option based on their personal values and preferences.

Tools for Enhancing Patient Engagement and Autonomy

Digital Health Technologies: Empowering Patients with Real-Time Data

Wearables and mobile health apps are revolutionising the way patients engage with their health. Devices that track heart rate, activity levels, sleep patterns, and other vital signs provide patients with real-time data, allowing them to monitor their health trends and make informed decisions about their lifestyle. These tools can also alert patients and healthcare providers to changes in health status, enabling early intervention.

A study published in the *Journal of Medical Internet Research* (2019) found that heart disease patients who used mobile health apps to track their health metrics were more likely to adhere to medication, engage in regular physical activity, and report higher levels of satisfaction with their care. Digital health technologies thus serve as valuable tools for patient empowerment, providing individuals with the information they need to take control of their health.

Telehealth Platforms: Expanding Access and Continuity of Care

Telehealth platforms facilitate remote consultations, follow-ups, and patient education, making healthcare more accessible and consistent. This is particularly beneficial for patients with chronic conditions like CAD, who require ongoing management and support. Through telehealth, patients can have regular check-ins with their healthcare providers, receive guidance on lifestyle modifications, and discuss any concerns related to their treatment plan without the need for in-person visits.

Telehealth has been shown to improve patient engagement and outcomes in cardiovascular care. A study published in *Circulation* (2020) found that patients with heart failure who participated in telehealth programs had fewer hospitalisations and emergency room visits compared to those receiving standard care. This suggests that telehealth can be an effective tool for enhancing patient engagement and maintaining continuity of care in chronic disease management.

Personal Health Records (PHR): Centralising Health Information

PHRs allow patients to access and manage their health information online. These tools help patients track their medical history, test results, and treatment plans, empowering them to manage their health proactively. PHRs can also be integrated with decision aids, educational resources, and appointment scheduling, making them a comprehensive platform for patient engagement.

The use of PHRs has been associated with improved health outcomes in chronic disease management. A study in the *American Journal of Managed Care* (2017) found that heart disease patients who used PHRs were more likely to adhere to treatment plans, attend follow-up appointments, and engage in preventive health behaviours. By centralising health information and making it accessible, PHRs enhance patient autonomy and facilitate informed decision-making.

Strategies for Effective Communication: Enhancing Understanding and Engagement

Cultural Competence and Health Literacy

Healthcare providers must be culturally competent to ensure that they can effectively communicate with and support patients from diverse backgrounds. This involves understanding and respecting cultural differences in values, beliefs, and behaviours related to health and disease. In cardiology, where lifestyle factors such as diet and exercise are critical, cultural competence is particularly important. Providers must be able to tailor recommendations to the patient's cultural context and preferences to enhance adherence and effectiveness.

Improving health literacy is another crucial aspect of patient-centred care. Providers must ensure that all communication is clear and accessible, avoiding medical jargon to minimise misunderstandings and help patients make informed decisions. Low health literacy has been linked to poorer health outcomes and higher rates of hospitalisation, particularly in chronic disease management. Strategies such as using visual aids, simplifying language, and verifying patient understanding through the "teach-back" method can improve health literacy and empower patients.

Empowering Patients through Lifestyle Changes

Educational Workshops and Support Groups: Building a Community of Care

Hospitals and health centres often offer workshops on nutrition, exercise, and stress management specifically tailored for cardiac patients. These workshops provide practical advice and support, helping patients implement and sustain lifestyle changes. Support groups also offer a platform for patients to share their experiences, challenges, and successes, fostering a sense of community and shared purpose.

Case studies have shown that participation in educational workshops can lead to significant improvements in heart health. For example, a patient named Emma, who had a history of heart disease, participated in a nutrition workshop that introduced her to the Mediterranean diet. With the support of her healthcare team and fellow workshop participants, Emma adopted the diet and, over time, experienced significant improvements in her cholesterol levels and overall heart health. This case underscores the value of educational support in empowering patient choices and promoting positive health outcomes.

Integrating Exercise and Stress Management into Care Plans

Physical activity and stress management are critical components of heart health. Providers can empower patients by helping them integrate these practices into their daily routines. Personalised exercise plans, yoga, meditation, and guided relaxation techniques can all be incorporated into the patient's care plan. These practices not only improve physical health but also enhance emotional well-being, reducing the risk of adverse cardiac events.

A study in *Psychosomatic Medicine* (2018) found that heart disease patients who participated in yoga and mindfulness-based stress reduction programs had lower levels of anxiety and depression, improved heart rate variability, and fewer hospitalisations compared to those receiving standard care. This evidence supports the inclusion of mind-body practices in cardiac care to empower patients and improve outcomes.

Dr Malhotra's Advocacy for Lifestyle-First Approaches

Dr Aseem Malhotra has been a strong proponent of lifestyle-first approaches in managing cardiovascular health. He argues that the overreliance on pharmacological interventions has led to a neglect of the root causes of heart disease, such as poor diet, physical inactivity, and chronic stress. Malhotra's advocacy is based on his clinical experience and research, which show that lifestyle interventions can be more effective than medications in certain populations.

In his book *The Pioppi Diet* and his numerous public health campaigns, Dr Malhotra emphasises the importance of empowering patients with the knowledge and tools to make healthier lifestyle choices. He encourages shared decision-making and informed consent, particularly in the context of statin therapy. His approach aligns with the principles of patient-centred care, which prioritise patient autonomy and the integration of evidence-based lifestyle interventions in chronic disease management.

Conclusion

Patient-centred care transforms patients from passive recipients of healthcare to active participants in their journey towards health. By emphasising education, shared decision-making, and the use of innovative tools, this approach enhances patient autonomy and improves health outcomes. The inclusion of advocates like Dr Aseem Malhotra, who champions transparency and lifestyle-based interventions, further strengthens the case for patient-centred care in cardiology. As healthcare continues to evolve, the focus will increasingly shift towards strategies that not only treat illness but also empower patients to maintain and enhance their health through informed, conscious choices.

Summary: Patient-Centred Care: Empowering Choices

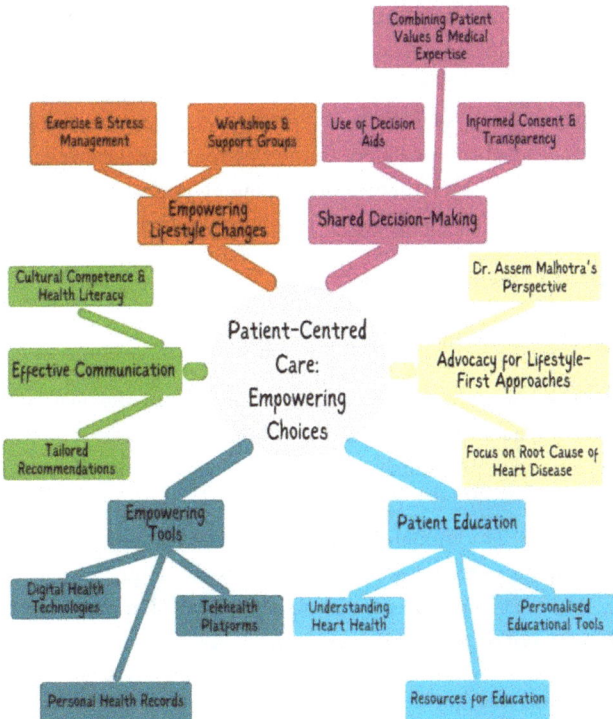

Chapter 9
Regulatory and Ethical Considerations

Introduction

The realm of cardiac care is undergoing a paradigm shift, with an increasing focus on integrating non-pharmacological and holistic approaches into mainstream treatment plans. However, despite the promising outcomes associated with these interventions, there are significant ethical, legal, and regulatory challenges that impede their widespread adoption. This chapter delves into these considerations, exploring the factors that influence the acceptance of non-pharmacological treatments in cardiology. By addressing these challenges head-on, we can pave the way for more balanced, patient-centred cardiac care that respects patient autonomy and ensures equitable access to all effective treatment options.

Ethical Considerations

1. Patient Autonomy and Informed Consent

Patient autonomy is a cornerstone of ethical medical practice. Respecting a patient's right to make informed decisions about their care involves providing comprehensive information about all available treatment options, including non-pharmacological alternatives. Traditionally, medical practice has leaned towards pharmaceutical and surgical interventions, sometimes neglecting to fully present lifestyle-based or holistic options that may align better with a patient's values and preferences.

One of the key ethical issues in cardiac care is ensuring that patients are given the opportunity to choose non-pharmacological interventions when appropriate. This involves a nuanced discussion of the benefits, risks, and limitations of each option, as well as the potential for non-pharmacological treatments to complement or even replace conventional therapies. For example, a patient with early-stage hypertension should be informed about the potential effectiveness of dietary changes, physical activity, and stress management techniques before being automatically prescribed antihypertensive medications.

Informed Consent and Shared Decision-Making:

Informed consent goes beyond simply presenting treatment options—it requires that patients fully understand the implications of each choice. Shared decision-making, where healthcare providers collaborate with patients to reach decisions that reflect the patient's values and preferences, is crucial. This approach not only enhances patient satisfaction but also improves adherence to treatment plans, as patients are more likely to engage with therapies they feel ownership over.

However, achieving true informed consent can be challenging in a healthcare environment where non-pharmacological interventions are often overshadowed by well-established pharmacological treatments. Addressing this imbalance requires a commitment from healthcare providers to present a complete picture of all available therapies supported by up-to-date, evidence-based information.

2. Equity and Access

Access to various treatment options is another ethical consideration in cardiac care. Socioeconomic disparities, geographical barriers, and healthcare system limitations often mean that non-pharmacological treatments, such as specialised dietary counselling, exercise programs, or stress management workshops, are less accessible to those in lower-income brackets or rural areas. This lack of access perpetuates health inequities and restricts the effectiveness of healthcare interventions at the population level.

Addressing Disparities:

To address these disparities, it is essential to advocate for policies that ensure equitable access to all effective treatments, regardless of socioeconomic status or geographical location. This might involve advocating for insurance coverage of lifestyle-based therapies, subsidising community health programs that offer non-pharmacological interventions, and ensuring that primary care providers are trained to implement and recommend these therapies as part of routine care.

Legal Considerations

1. Regulation of Non-Pharmacological Treatments

One of the major legal challenges facing non-pharmacological interventions is the lack of standardised regulatory frameworks. Unlike pharmaceutical treatments, which undergo rigorous testing and approval processes, many non-pharmacological therapies do not have the same level of regulation, leading to variability in quality, safety, and efficacy.

Call for Standardisation:

Establishing robust regulatory standards for non-pharmacological interventions, including natural supplements, herbal therapies, and alternative treatments, is necessary to enhance their credibility and ensure patient safety. This may involve creating certification programs for practitioners of non-pharmacological therapies, setting guidelines for the manufacture and distribution of supplements, and implementing regulatory oversight to monitor adverse effects.

2. Liability Issues

Healthcare providers who recommend non-pharmacological treatments may face legal liabilities, particularly if these treatments are perceived as deviating from conventional medical standards. Concerns about malpractice and the potential for litigation can deter clinicians from recommending non-pharmacological options, even when these may be appropriate for certain patients.

Developing Clear Guidelines:

To address these concerns, it is important to develop clear clinical guidelines and protocols for the use of non-pharmacological treatments in cardiac care. These guidelines should be based on the best available evidence and should outline appropriate contexts for recommending such treatments. Additionally, healthcare providers should be encouraged to document patient discussions and decisions thoroughly to demonstrate that informed consent was obtained and that non-pharmacological options were presented as part of a comprehensive treatment plan.

Regulatory Challenges

1. Integration into Standard Care

Integrating non-pharmacological treatments into standard medical practice presents several challenges, including resistance from the medical community, lack of support from insurance providers, and limited training in medical education. Many healthcare professionals receive little to no formal education on lifestyle-based therapies or complementary and alternative medicine (CAM), leading to a lack of familiarity and confidence in recommending these approaches.

Educational Initiatives:

To overcome these barriers, medical schools and continuing education programs should incorporate training on the science and application of non-pharmacological interventions. This would empower healthcare providers to feel more confident in discussing and recommending these therapies to patients. Additionally, fostering collaborations between conventional and CAM practitioners can facilitate knowledge exchange and integration of diverse treatment modalities.

2. Insurance and Reimbursement

One of the most significant barriers to the adoption of non-pharmacological treatments is the lack of insurance coverage. Many insurance plans cover pharmaceutical and surgical treatments but exclude lifestyle-based therapies, nutritional counselling, and other holistic interventions. This discrepancy creates a financial disincentive for both patients and providers to pursue non-pharmacological options, even when these may be more cost-effective and beneficial in the long run.

Advocating for Policy Change:

To promote the broader adoption of non-pharmacological therapies, policy changes are needed that recognise the cost-effectiveness and therapeutic value of these interventions. This could involve lobbying for the inclusion of evidence-based lifestyle and complementary therapies in insurance coverage, establishing reimbursement codes for non-pharmacological treatments, and demonstrating the potential for these therapies to reduce long-term healthcare costs.

Addressing Systemic Biases

1. Promotion of Pharmacological Treatments

The pharmaceutical industry exerts a powerful influence on medical practice and research. This influence often manifests in the promotion of drug therapies at the expense of non-pharmacological approaches. Pharmaceutical companies fund a substantial portion of clinical research, sponsor continuing medical education programs, and contribute to the development of clinical guidelines. As a result, treatment recommendations may disproportionately favour pharmacological solutions, even in cases where non-pharmacological interventions could be equally effective.

Towards a Balanced Approach:

To counteract this imbalance, it is essential to promote a more balanced approach that gives equal weight to non-pharmacological methods. This could involve creating funding mechanisms for research into non-pharmacological therapies, ensuring transparency in guideline development, and fostering collaborations between academic institutions and practitioners of holistic medicine.

2. Research and Evidence

Non-pharmacological treatments often suffer from a lack of high-quality research due to limited funding and the challenges associated with studying complex lifestyle interventions. This creates a cycle where insufficient evidence prevents the adoption of these therapies, which in turn limits further research opportunities.

Promoting Rigorous Research:

To break this cycle, increased research funding is needed to evaluate non-pharmacological treatments using rigorous scientific methods. This could include randomised controlled trials (RCTs) where feasible, as well as other research designs such as observational studies, cohort studies, and systematic reviews. Establishing centres of excellence for research in integrative medicine can also help build the evidence base necessary to support the inclusion of these therapies in mainstream practice.

The Limits of Randomised Controlled Trials

While RCTs are considered the gold standard for evaluating medical interventions, they have limitations when it comes to assessing non-pharmacological treatments. Issues such as cost, ethical constraints, and the difficulty of blinding participants to lifestyle interventions can make RCTs impractical for studying holistic approaches. Furthermore, RCTs often exclude diverse populations and comorbidities, limiting the generalisability of their findings.

Alternative Research Approaches:

Recognising the limitations of RCTs, there is a need for a diverse range of research designs to comprehensively evaluate the efficacy of non-pharmacological treatments. Pragmatic trials, which study interventions in real-world settings, and qualitative research, which explores patient experiences and outcomes, can provide valuable insights that complement the findings of RCTs.

Conclusion

The future of cardiac care lies in embracing a model that equally values pharmacological and non-pharmacological treatments. This shift requires overcoming regulatory, legal, and ethical challenges to create a healthcare environment that supports comprehensive and integrative care options. By advocating for policies that ensure equitable access, promoting rigorous research into holistic therapies, and addressing systemic biases within the medical community, we can foster a more balanced approach to cardiac care. Such a transformation will enable patients to benefit from a wider range of effective therapies and will ultimately contribute to better health outcomes and quality of life.

The integration of non-pharmacological innovations into mainstream cardiac care is not only feasible but necessary. With proper regulatory support, ethical practices, and robust evidence, we can move towards a future where patients have access to all effective treatment options, empowering them to achieve optimal heart health.

Summary: Regulatory and Ethical Considerations

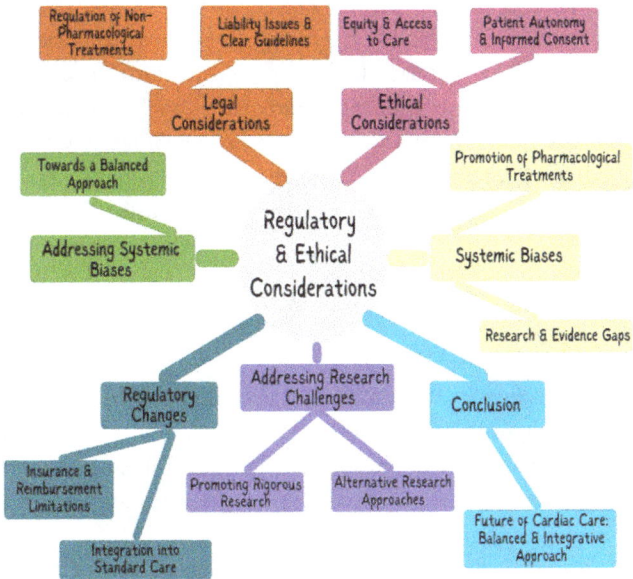

Chapter 10
Revitalising the Heart

The Role of IV Therapies in Cardiac Regeneration

Introduction

Intravenous (IV) therapies are emerging as potent adjuncts in the management of cardiac health, complementing conventional treatments with potential regenerative capabilities. This chapter explores the integration of IV therapies like glutathione, Vitamin C, and other micronutrients, including the critical role of Nicotinamide Adenine Dinucleotide (NAD+), in supporting cardiac function and overall heart health.

Overview of IV Therapies in Cardiology IV Therapies Explained

IV therapies involve the administration of nutrients directly into the bloodstream, offering higher concentrations and immediate availability compared to oral supplements. This method ensures that nutrients bypass the digestive system, where absorption can sometimes be compromised.

Common IV Therapies for Cardiac Health

Vitamin C:

Known for its antioxidant properties, high doses of Vitamin C administered intravenously can combat oxidative stress, a key factor in heart disease.

Glutathione:

Often referred to as the body's 'master antioxidant,' glutathione plays a crucial role in reducing oxidative stress and inflammation within the cardiovascular system.

Magnesium:

Essential for heart health, IV magnesium can help regulate heart rhythm, lower blood pressure, and improve endothelial function.

NAD+:

A coenzyme involved in hundreds of metabolic processes, including energy production and DNA repair. NAD+ levels decline with age, and boosting these levels can potentially rejuvenate cells and support heart health.

Scientific Evidence and Clinical Studies Research Findings:

Studies have shown that high-dose IV Vitamin C reduces inflammatory markers associated with heart disease. Clinical trials involving IV magnesium have demonstrated its effectiveness in treating arrhythmias and improving outcomes in patients with congestive heart failure. Emerging research suggests that NAD+ therapies can help restore cellular function and reduce oxidative stress, potentially benefiting heart health.

Mechanisms of Action:

Antioxidants like Vitamin C and glutathione neutralise free radicals, reducing oxidative damage to cardiac cells and vascular tissues. Magnesium acts as a natural calcium channel blocker, which helps dilate blood vessels, improving blood flow and reducing the workload on the heart. NAD+ plays a crucial role in cellular energy metabolism and may help improve the function of mitochondria within heart cells, promoting better cardiac performance.

Case Studies and Patient Testimonials Patient Experiences:

Case Study 1:

A patient with chronic heart failure experienced significant improvement in symptoms and quality of life after receiving a series of glutathione IV treatments.

Case Study 2:

Another patient, suffering from post-myocardial infarction fatigue, reported enhanced energy levels and overall well-being following high-dose IV Vitamin C therapy.

Case Study 3:

A recent case involving NAD+ therapy showed a patient with age-related cardiac dysfunction experiencing improved cardiac output and reduced symptoms of heart fatigue.

Integration into Cardiac Care Combining IV Therapies with Conventional Treatments:

IV therapies are best used in conjunction with lifestyle changes and standard medical treatments. This integrative approach can maximise heart health and potentially speed up recovery processes. Protocols for incorporating IV therapies should be tailored to individual patient needs, based on specific cardiac conditions and overall health profiles.

Regulatory and Safety Considerations Ensuring Safety:

While IV therapies are generally safe, they must be administered under medical supervision to avoid complications such as infections or imbalances in electrolytes. Regulatory oversight is crucial to ensure the quality and safety of substances used in IV therapies.

Ethical and Legal Implications:

Practitioners must obtain informed consent, explaining the potential benefits and risks associated with IV therapies. Patients should be fully aware of their treatment options and the relative experimental nature of some IV therapies in cardiology.

Conclusion

IV therapies offer exciting possibilities in the realm of cardiac care, providing supportive treatment that can enhance the efficacy of traditional therapies and contribute to heart health regeneration. As research continues to evolve, these therapies may become more mainstream, offering patients innovative options to manage and potentially improve their cardiovascular health. With proper oversight, informed consent, and integration into comprehensive treatment plans, IV therapies hold the potential to make significant contributions to the field of cardiology.

Summary: Revitalising the Heart

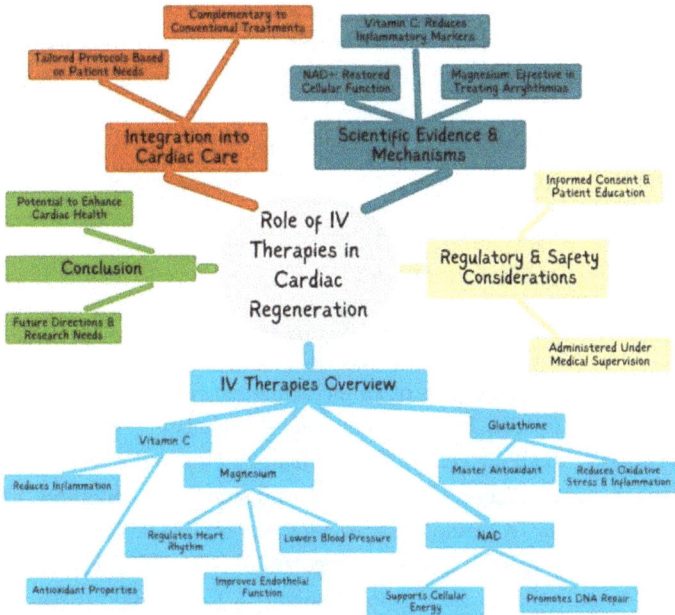

Chapter 11
Nature's Bounty: Peptides and Herbs for Heart Health

Introduction

The prevalence of cardiovascular disease (CVD) has reached alarming levels worldwide, prompting healthcare professionals to explore new and innovative treatment strategies. While conventional pharmacological approaches have been instrumental in reducing mortality and managing symptoms, there is an increasing interest in integrating natural therapies, such as peptides and herbs, into cardiac care. This chapter delves into the role of these natural compounds in enhancing cardiovascular health, supported by scientific research and traditional uses. By understanding how peptides and herbs work in synergy with conventional treatments, healthcare providers can offer patients a comprehensive, Personalised approach that leverages the best of both worlds.

Peptides in Cardiac Health

Overview of Cardiac Peptides

Peptides are short chains of amino acids that function as signalling molecules in the body. Their role in regulating physiological processes, such as cell growth, inflammation, and tissue repair, makes them ideal candidates for addressing complex conditions like heart disease. In cardiology, peptides can influence key pathways involved in blood pressure regulation, vascular health, and myocardial repair, offering novel solutions for conditions that are traditionally managed with pharmacological agents alone.

Peptides are synthesised in the body in response to various stimuli and can either exert local effects or enter the bloodstream to act on distant organs. For instance, natriuretic peptides produced by the heart regulate blood pressure and fluid balance, while thymosins, primarily known for their immunomodulatory properties, have demonstrated benefits in cardiac tissue repair. This versatility has propelled the research and development of synthetic peptides and peptide analogues that can target specific aspects of cardiovascular health, such as reducing inflammation or promoting angiogenesis.

Specific Peptides for Heart Health

1. **B-type Natriuretic Peptide (BNP)**: BNP is released by the heart in response to excessive stretching of the heart muscles, often seen in conditions like heart failure. It acts by promoting diuresis (the excretion of water and sodium) and vasodilation, which decreases blood volume and reduces the workload on the heart. Clinically, elevated BNP levels are used as a diagnostic and prognostic marker for heart failure. BNP analogues, such as Nesiritide, have been developed to mimic these effects and are used in acute heart failure management to alleviate symptoms and improve hemodynamics.

The therapeutic use of BNP and its analogues has shown promise in reducing hospital readmission rates for heart failure patients and improving quality of life. However, the application of BNP therapy requires careful monitoring, as excessive diuresis or vasodilation can lead to adverse effects like hypotension.

2. **Vascular Endothelial Growth Factor (VEGF)**: VEGF is a potent angiogenic peptide that stimulates the formation of new blood vessels. This process is crucial in ischemic heart diseases, where the blood supply to the heart is compromised. By promoting angiogenesis, VEGF helps restore oxygen supply to ischemic tissues, reducing symptoms such as angina and improving myocardial function.

VEGF therapies are currently being explored in clinical trials for their potential to treat refractory angina and peripheral artery disease. Early results are promising, showing enhanced perfusion to ischemic areas and improved patient outcomes. Future research is focused on optimising the delivery of VEGF to target tissues and minimising systemic side effects.

3. **Thymosin Beta-4 (TB4)**: Thymosin Beta-4 is a naturally occurring peptide that has gained attention for its regenerative properties. Following myocardial infarction (heart attack), TB4 has been shown to promote cell migration, survival, and differentiation, which are essential for tissue repair. Preclinical studies have demonstrated that TB4 can reduce scar formation, increase angiogenesis, and improve overall cardiac function post-infarction.

In clinical settings, TB4 is being investigated as a potential adjunctive therapy for cardiac repair. Its ability to modulate the inflammatory response and reduce fibrosis holds promise for enhancing recovery in patients with ischemic heart disease and other forms of cardiac injury.

4. **Angiotensin-(1-7)**: Angiotensin-(1-7) is a peptide fragment of the renin-angiotensin-aldosterone system (RAAS) that exerts counter-regulatory effects against the traditional RAAS pathway, which promotes vasoconstriction and sodium retention. By activating the Mas receptor, Angiotensin-(1-7) induces vasodilation, reduces blood pressure, and has been shown to exhibit anti-inflammatory and antifibrotic properties. Research has suggested its potential use in treating hypertension and heart failure, particularly in patients who do not respond well to conventional RAAS inhibitors like ACE inhibitors and ARBs.

The therapeutic potential of Angiotensin-(1-7) lies in its ability to modulate the deleterious effects of angiotensin II while preserving the beneficial effects of the RAAS pathway, offering a nuanced approach to managing cardiovascular conditions.

Herbal Therapies in Cardiology

Role of Traditional Herbs

For centuries, herbs have been a cornerstone of traditional medicine for managing heart health. Many herbs contain bioactive compounds that exert antioxidant, anti-inflammatory, lipid-lowering, and vasodilatory effects, making them valuable adjuncts to conventional cardiac treatments. Modern scientific research has begun to elucidate the mechanisms through which these herbs confer their benefits, validating their traditional use and paving the way for their integration into evidence-based cardiac care.

Incorporating herbal therapies into cardiology is not without challenges. Variability in herb quality, potency, and standardisation can affect therapeutic outcomes. Therefore, it is essential to use standardised extracts with known concentrations of active constituents to achieve consistent and reliable results. Additionally, understanding the potential interactions between herbs and conventional medications is crucial to avoid adverse effects.

Key Herbs for Cardiac Care

1. **Hawthorn (Crataegus spp.)**: Hawthorn is often referred to as the "heart herb" due to its long-standing use in supporting cardiac function. It contains a variety of bioactive compounds, including flavonoids and procyanidins, which have been shown to improve coronary blood flow, reduce myocardial oxygen consumption, and strengthen heart contractions. Clinical studies have demonstrated that hawthorn extract can reduce symptoms of heart failure, such as fatigue and dyspnea, and improve exercise tolerance.

Hawthorn's cardioprotective effects are thought to be mediated through its antioxidant activity and its ability to modulate nitric oxide, a key regulator of vascular tone. As a result, hawthorn is often recommended for patients with mild to moderate heart failure or as a preventive measure for those at risk of cardiovascular disease.

2. **Garlic (Allium sativum):** Garlic is one of the most extensively researched herbs for cardiovascular health. Its active component, allicin, is responsible for many of its therapeutic effects, including lowering blood pressure, reducing cholesterol, and inhibiting platelet aggregation. A meta-analysis published in the *Journal of Clinical Hypertension* found that garlic supplementation could reduce systolic and diastolic blood pressure by an average of 8.4 mmHg and 7.3 mmHg, respectively, in hypertensive patients.

Beyond its antihypertensive effects, garlic has been shown to reduce LDL cholesterol and increase HDL cholesterol, further supporting its use as part of a comprehensive heart health regimen. Additionally, its ability to inhibit platelet aggregation makes it a valuable adjunct for preventing thromboembolic events in patients with coronary artery disease.

3. **Arjuna (Terminalia arjuna):** Arjuna is a prominent herb in Ayurvedic medicine known for its cardiotonic and antioxidant properties. Studies have shown that arjuna bark extract can improve cardiac output, reduce blood pressure, and enhance the overall function of the heart. Its cardioprotective effects are attributed to its rich phytochemical content, which includes tannins, glycosides, and flavonoids.

Research published in *Phytotherapy Research* demonstrated that arjuna supplementation reduced the frequency and severity of angina episodes in patients with chronic stable angina. Furthermore, it improved left ventricular function, suggesting its potential as a supportive therapy for heart failure and ischemic heart disease.

4. **Turmeric (Curcuma longa):** Curcumin, the active compound in turmeric, is a potent anti-inflammatory and antioxidant agent. It has been shown to modulate inflammatory pathways, reduce oxidative stress, and improve endothelial function, all of which are critical factors in the pathogenesis of atherosclerosis and other cardiovascular diseases.

A study in *Nutrition Journal* reported that curcumin supplementation significantly reduced markers of systemic inflammation, such as C-reactive protein (CRP), in patients with metabolic syndrome. This reduction in inflammation translates into improved vascular health and a lower risk of cardiovascular events, making curcumin a valuable herb for heart health.

5. **Ginkgo Biloba**: Ginkgo biloba has traditionally been used to enhance circulation and cognitive function, but its benefits extend to cardiovascular health as well. Ginkgo's vasodilatory effects, mediated through its influence on nitric oxide pathways, can help improve blood flow and reduce the risk of thrombus formation.

Clinical studies have indicated that ginkgo supplementation can improve peripheral circulation, making it beneficial for patients with intermittent claudication and other peripheral vascular conditions. Additionally, its antioxidant properties help protect against oxidative damage to blood vessels, contributing to overall cardiovascular health.

Clinical Studies and Evidence

A wealth of scientific literature supports the use of peptides and herbs in managing cardiovascular conditions. For example, a double-blind, placebo-controlled trial involving hawthorn extract showed significant improvements in cardiac output and reduced symptoms of heart failure compared to placebo. Similarly, clinical trials on garlic have demonstrated its efficacy in lowering blood pressure and cholesterol levels, highlighting its potential as a natural adjunct to antihypertensive and lipid-lowering medications.

The therapeutic potential of peptides is also being explored in clinical trials. Studies on BNP analogues have shown their ability to reduce hospital readmission rates in heart failure patients, while VEGF and TB4 therapies are being evaluated for their regenerative effects in ischemic heart disease and myocardial infarction recovery.

Integrating Peptides and Herbs into Cardiac Care

The integration of peptides and herbal therapies into cardiac care requires careful consideration of dosing, quality control, and potential interactions with conventional medications. Healthcare providers should work closely with patients to tailor treatment regimens that incorporate these natural agents without compromising safety or efficacy.

Regulatory Aspects and Future Directions

The regulatory landscape for peptide and herbal therapies is complex, with varying standards across different regions. Ensuring the safety and efficacy of these therapies requires rigorous quality control, standardised extraction methods, and comprehensive clinical trials. As the field of integrative cardiology continues to evolve, collaboration between traditional healers, herbalists, and modern medical practitioners will be essential to bridge the gap between traditional knowledge and contemporary scientific validation.

Conclusion

Peptides and herbal therapies offer a promising complementary approach to conventional cardiac care. With their ability to modulate key physiological processes and improve cardiovascular function, these natural agents have the potential to enhance patient outcomes and reduce reliance on pharmacological treatments. As research continues to uncover the full extent of their benefits, peptides like BNP and TB4, along with herbs like hawthorn, garlic, arjuna, and turmeric, will likely become integral components of holistic cardiac health management. The future of cardiology lies in harnessing nature's wisdom and modern science to provide patients with comprehensive care that nurtures the heart and promotes overall well-being.

Summary: Nature's Bounty: Peptides and Herbs for Heart Health

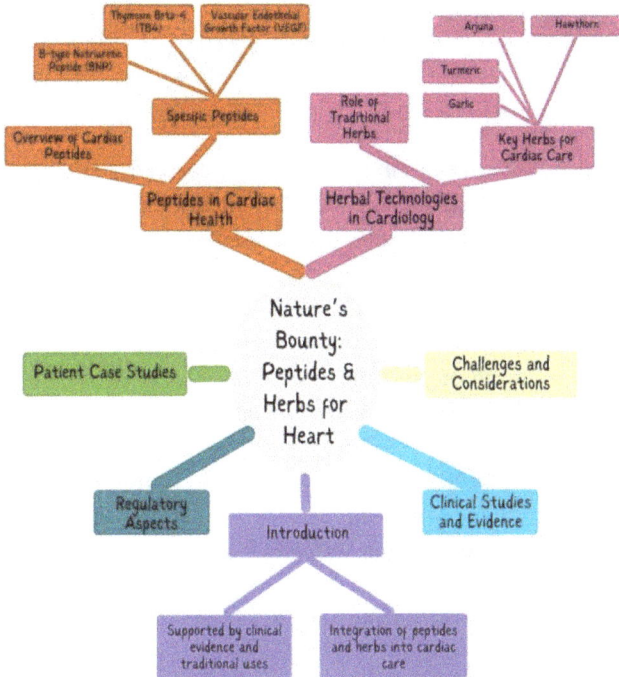

Chapter 12
Beyond the Heartbeat: Vasomotor Control of Circulation

Introduction

Vasomotor control of circulation plays a crucial role in regulating blood flow and maintaining blood pressure, which are vital for overall cardiovascular health. The vasomotor system, governed by the autonomic nervous system, adjusts the diameter of blood vessels, thereby influencing resistance and blood flow throughout the circulatory system. Dysfunctions in vasomotor control can lead to hypertension and other cardiovascular disorders, contributing to an increased risk of morbidity and mortality. This chapter explores the non-pharmacological methods—such as temperature therapy, breathwork, controlled physical exercise, and diet—that influence vasomotor function to improve circulatory health, backed by scientific evidence and clinical studies.

Understanding Vasomotor Control

Vasomotor Basics

The term "vasomotor" refers to the processes that regulate the contraction and relaxation of blood vessel walls through the autonomic nervous system, primarily the sympathetic and parasympathetic branches. The vasomotor centre, located in the medulla oblongata of the brainstem, integrates sensory input from baroreceptors and chemoreceptors to modulate blood vessel tone. Vasoconstriction and vasodilation, mediated by neurotransmitters such as norepinephrine and acetylcholine, respectively, are the primary mechanisms through which blood flow is regulated.

- **Sympathetic Nervous System:** Activation of the sympathetic nervous system releases norepinephrine, leading to vasoconstriction, which increases vascular resistance and raises blood pressure. This response is crucial during activities that demand increased blood flow, such as exercise or the fight-or-flight response.

- **Parasympathetic Nervous System:** Conversely, activation of the parasympathetic nervous system through the release of acetylcholine induces vasodilation, which decreases vascular resistance and lowers blood pressure, promoting a state of relaxation and improved circulation to vital organs.

Significance in Cardiac Health

Proper vasomotor function ensures adequate blood supply to the heart, brain, and other vital organs. Dysfunctions in this system can lead to conditions such as hypertension, atherosclerosis, and endothelial dysfunction—all of which are major risk factors for cardiovascular diseases. Endothelial cells, which line the inner surface of blood vessels, play a pivotal role in maintaining vascular tone by releasing vasodilators like nitric oxide (NO) and vasoconstrictors like endothelin. Any imbalance in these mechanisms can disrupt blood flow and promote the development of cardiovascular pathology.

Non-Pharmacological Methods to Enhance Vasomotor Function

Temperature Therapy

1. Cold Exposure:

Brief exposures to cold, such as cold-water immersion, ice baths, or cryotherapy, can enhance vasomotor response by inducing vasoconstriction followed by reflexive vasodilation upon rewarming. This alternating vascular response strengthens blood vessel walls and improves overall vascular reactivity. Cold exposure has been shown to increase levels of norepinephrine and reduce inflammation, contributing to improved blood flow and heart rate variability (HRV).

- **Scientific Evidence:** A study published in the *European Journal of Applied Physiology* (2018) investigated the effects of cold-water immersion on cardiovascular function and found that regular exposure led to improved endothelial function and enhanced arterial compliance in healthy individuals. These changes were attributed to increased nitric oxide bioavailability and reduced oxidative stress.

2. Heat Therapy:

Heat therapy, including sauna use and hot baths, induces heat stress that promotes vasodilation, thereby improving circulation and arterial compliance. The heat increases blood flow to the skin and peripheral tissues, reduces vascular resistance, and lowers blood pressure. Regular heat exposure has been associated with reduced cardiovascular mortality and lower risk of hypertension.

- **Scientific Evidence:** A longitudinal study published in *JAMA Internal Medicine* (2015) examined the effects of frequent sauna use in a cohort of Finnish men and found that those who used saunas 4-7 times per week had a 50% lower risk of fatal cardiovascular events compared to those who used saunas once a week. The study attributed these benefits to improved vascular function and reduced oxidative stress markers.

Breathwork and Vasomotor Function

Breathwork techniques, such as slow breathing and diaphragmatic breathing, influence vasomotor control by modulating autonomic nervous system activity. Slow breathing has been shown to enhance baroreflex sensitivity, which regulates blood pressure in response to changes in blood vessel stretch.

- **Scientific Evidence:** A study published in *Hypertension* (2013) demonstrated that participants who engaged in slow breathing (six breaths per minute) for 15 minutes daily experienced significant reductions in blood pressure and an increase in HRV. The study suggested that slow breathing activates the parasympathetic nervous system, leading to enhanced vasodilation and improved vasomotor control.

Controlled Physical Exercise

1. Endurance Training:

Regular aerobic exercise, such as walking, cycling, or swimming, enhances endothelial function and vasomotor responsiveness by increasing the bioavailability of nitric oxide (NO), a crucial mediator for vasodilation. NO is synthesised by endothelial cells in response to shear stress induced by increased blood flow during exercise. This molecule relaxes the smooth muscle in blood vessel walls, promoting vasodilation and improving blood flow.

- **Scientific Evidence:** A meta-analysis published in *Circulation* (2016) reviewed the effects of aerobic exercise on vascular function and found that regular aerobic activity significantly improved endothelial-dependent vasodilation and decreased arterial stiffness in both healthy individuals and patients with cardiovascular risk factors.

2. Resistance Training:

Moderate resistance training has been proven to improve vascular function by inducing growth factors that help maintain healthy blood vessels. Resistance training also increases the density of capillaries in skeletal muscles, improving oxygen delivery and overall cardiovascular efficiency.

- **Scientific Evidence:** A study in the *American Journal of Physiology* (2012) reported that resistance training improved endothelial function and increased the production of vascular endothelial growth factor (VEGF), which promotes the formation of new blood vessels and enhances circulation.

Dietary Interventions and Vasomotor Control

Dietary choices have a profound impact on vasomotor function. Diets rich in antioxidants, nitrates, and polyphenols have been shown to enhance endothelial function and improve vasomotor responsiveness.

- **Nitrates:** Found abundantly in leafy greens like spinach and beets, nitrates are converted to nitric oxide in the body, which enhances vasodilation and blood flow. A study published in *Hypertension* (2013) found that dietary nitrate supplementation improved endothelial function and reduced blood pressure in hypertensive patients.

- **Polyphenols:** Present in foods like berries, dark chocolate, and red wine, polyphenols have been shown to enhance nitric oxide synthesis and reduce oxidative stress, contributing to improved vascular health. A review in *Nutrients* (2017) highlighted that regular consumption of polyphenol-rich foods is associated with improved arterial compliance and reduced risk of cardiovascular events.

Integrating Vasomotor Control in Cardiac Rehabilitation

Cardiac rehabilitation programs increasingly incorporate elements that target vasomotor health, including tailored exercise routines, breathwork, and temperature therapies. These programs are designed to help patients recover from cardiac events and surgeries and to maintain long-term cardiovascular health.

- **Exercise Prescription:** Cardiac rehabilitation often includes both aerobic and resistance training to improve vasomotor control. These programs are individualised based on the patient's health status and exercise capacity, ensuring safety and effectiveness.

- **Temperature Therapy:** Incorporating sauna sessions or contrast baths (alternating hot and cold water immersion) into rehabilitation can improve vasomotor function and promote vascular health.

Case Studies and Clinical Evidence

Real-World Applications

Case Study 1:

A 55-year-old male patient with a history of hypertension and borderline endothelial dysfunction participated in a controlled study involving regular sauna sessions. After six weeks of using the sauna three times a week, his blood pressure dropped by 10/5 mmHg, and arterial stiffness, measured by pulse wave velocity, showed significant improvement. The patient also reported enhanced exercise tolerance and overall well-being.

Case Study 2:

A 60-year-old female patient recovering from myocardial infarction engaged in a structured aerobic and resistance training program as part of her cardiac rehabilitation. After 12 weeks, the patient showed marked improvement in endothelial function, as measured by flow-mediated dilation. Her heart rate variability also improved, indicating better autonomic control. The integration of slow breathing techniques further enhanced her cardiovascular function, demonstrating the synergistic benefits of combining different vasomotor control methods.

Challenges and Future Directions

Overcoming Challenges

Implementing these therapies requires careful medical supervision, especially for patients with severe cardiovascular conditions. Monitoring and adjustments based on individual responses are crucial for safety and effectiveness. Educating patients and healthcare providers about the benefits and techniques of vasomotor control therapies is essential for their wider acceptance and implementation.

Research is ongoing to better understand the precise mechanisms through which non-pharmacological methods influence vasomotor function. Future studies may focus on Personalised approaches that combine temperature therapy, exercise, and dietary interventions tailored to an individual's genetic and physiological profile.

Conclusion

Understanding and manipulating vasomotor control through non-pharmacological methods presents a promising avenue for enhancing circulatory health and managing cardiovascular diseases. As research continues to evolve, these methods could become integral components of preventive strategies and therapeutic interventions in cardiology. This holistic approach not only aids in immediate recovery and rehabilitation but also contributes to long-term cardiovascular health, providing patients with tools to actively manage their heart health. Through a combination of evidence-based strategies—such as temperature therapy, breathwork, exercise, and diet—patients can achieve optimal vasomotor function, thereby reducing the burden of cardiovascular diseases and improving overall quality of life.

Summary: Beyond the Heartbeat: Vasomotor Control of Circulation

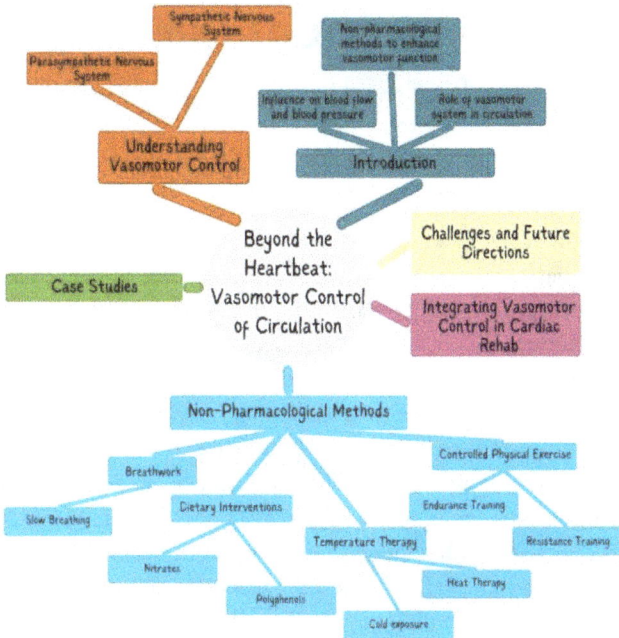

Chapter 13
Heart Health Myths: Aligning with Non-Pharmacological Interventions

Introduction

This chapter addresses prevalent myths in cardiology, particularly those that undermine the efficacy of non-pharmacological interventions like diet, exercise, mindfulness, and the management of inflammation, hormonal balance, and gut health. These misconceptions have often led to an over-reliance on pharmacological treatments, overlooking the powerful potential of holistic approaches to prevent and manage heart disease. By challenging these myths with scientific evidence, we aim to highlight the significant role of integrative strategies in promoting cardiovascular health. Understanding the truth behind these myths empowers patients and healthcare providers to make informed decisions that align with long-term heart health.

Myth 1: Diet and Exercise Can't Match Medications

Revised View:

Fact: Lifestyle interventions, when properly implemented, can be as effective as medications, particularly for preventing heart disease and improving overall cardiovascular health. In some cases, diet and exercise can not only prevent but also reverse certain heart conditions.

Supporting Evidence:

Numerous studies have demonstrated the effectiveness of diet and exercise in improving heart health outcomes. For instance, the Lyon

Diet Heart Study, a landmark clinical trial, demonstrated that individuals who adhered to a Mediterranean diet had a 72% lower risk of recurrent heart attacks and cardiovascular events compared to those on a standard post-infarction diet. This was achieved without additional pharmacological interventions, underscoring the power of diet in secondary prevention of heart disease.

Moreover, the **Ornish Lifestyle Medicine Program**, which includes a plant-based diet, regular physical activity, stress management techniques, and social support, has been shown to reverse severe coronary artery disease. A study published in the *Lancet* (1990) found that patients with severe CAD who followed this lifestyle program experienced regression of atherosclerotic plaques and improved myocardial perfusion, comparable to or even exceeding the outcomes seen with certain pharmacological and surgical interventions.

Myth 2: Heart Disease is Mostly About Genetics

Revised View:

Fact: While genetics do play a role in cardiovascular risk, lifestyle factors such as diet, physical activity, and stress management have a far greater impact on heart health. The majority of heart disease cases are influenced by modifiable risk factors.

Supporting Evidence:

The INTERHEART Study, a large-scale epidemiological study involving over 27,000 participants across multiple countries, found that approximately 90% of heart disease cases could be attributed to modifiable lifestyle factors, including unhealthy diet, lack of physical activity, smoking, and psychological stress. This highlights the potential of non-pharmacological interventions to prevent and manage heart conditions, even in individuals with a genetic predisposition.

Further evidence comes from research on epigenetics, which shows that lifestyle choices can influence gene expression related to cardiovascular health. For example, regular physical exercise has been shown to upregulate genes associated with antioxidant defence and anti-inflammatory pathways, providing a protective effect against cardiovascular disease.

Myth 3: Hormonal Treatments are Unrelated to Heart Health

Revised View:

Fact: Hormonal imbalances can significantly affect cardiovascular health, and optimising these hormones can improve heart function and reduce cardiovascular risk.

Supporting Evidence:

Hormonal imbalances, such as hypothyroidism or hyperthyroidism, are closely linked to cardiovascular dysfunctions. Hypothyroidism, for instance, can lead to increased cholesterol levels, bradycardia, and elevated diastolic blood pressure, all of which are risk factors for heart disease. Conversely, hyperthyroidism can increase heart rate and cardiac workload, predisposing patients to arrhythmias.

Sex hormones, such as oestrogen and testosterone, also play crucial roles in cardiovascular health. Oestrogen is known to have a protective effect on the vascular endothelium, promoting vasodilation and improving cholesterol metabolism. Postmenopausal women are at increased risk of heart disease due to the decline in oestrogen levels. Similarly, low testosterone levels in men have been linked to increased risk of cardiovascular events, highlighting the need for balanced hormonal management.

Clinical studies have shown that bioidentical hormone replacement therapy (BHRT) in women and testosterone replacement in men can improve lipid profiles, enhance endothelial function, and reduce inflammatory markers, thereby reducing overall cardiovascular risk.

Myth 4: Mindfulness and Stress Reduction Are Just Placebos

Revised View:

Fact: Mindfulness and stress reduction techniques have a direct impact on physiological parameters such as blood pressure, heart rate variability, and inflammatory markers, which are critical for heart health.

Supporting Evidence:

Mindfulness-based stress reduction (MBSR), meditation, and yoga have all been shown to influence cardiovascular health positively. A meta-analysis published in the *Journal of Hypertension* (2016) concluded that mindfulness practices reduce systolic and diastolic blood pressure, comparable to the effects of some antihypertensive medications. The mechanism involves activation of the parasympathetic nervous system, which lowers cortisol levels and reduces the stress response.

In addition, a study published in *Psychosomatic Medicine* (2018) found that individuals who practised meditation had significantly lower levels of C-reactive protein (CRP), a marker of systemic inflammation. Lower CRP levels are associated with reduced risk of atherosclerosis and coronary artery disease.

Mindfulness practices also improve heart rate variability (HRV), an indicator of autonomic nervous system balance. Higher HRV is linked to better cardiovascular resilience and reduced risk of sudden cardiac events.

Myth 5: Gut Health Has No Connection to Heart Health

Revised View:

Fact: The gut microbiome plays a crucial role in cardiovascular health by influencing systemic inflammation, cholesterol metabolism, and even the integrity of the vascular wall.

Supporting Evidence:

The gut-heart axis is an emerging area of research that highlights the interconnectedness of the gastrointestinal and cardiovascular systems. The gut microbiome produces metabolites such as trimethylamine N-oxide (TMAO), which has been implicated in the development of atherosclerosis. Elevated levels of TMAO are associated with an increased risk of heart attack, stroke, and cardiovascular mortality.

Dietary interventions that promote a healthy gut microbiome, such as high-fibre diets and probiotic supplementation, have been shown to lower TMAO levels and reduce systemic inflammation. A study published in *Nature Medicine* (2018) found that individuals with a diverse gut microbiome had lower levels of inflammatory markers and improved endothelial function compared to those with less diverse microbial populations.

Moreover, the Mediterranean diet, rich in fibre, polyphenols, and healthy fats, has been shown to favourably alter the gut microbiome, leading to reduced cardiovascular risk. This underscores the importance of gut health in the context of heart disease prevention and management.

Conclusion

Dispelling these myths emphasises the effectiveness and importance of non-pharmacological interventions in cardiac care. By incorporating holistic approaches that address lifestyle, diet, mindfulness, hormonal balance, and gut health, patients and healthcare providers can work together towards more effective prevention and management of heart disease. This chapter aims to realign perceptions towards embracing and integrating comprehensive, evidence-based strategies for enhancing heart health without solely relying on medications. As more research supports the interconnectedness of body systems, it becomes clear that a multifaceted approach is not only beneficial but necessary for achieving optimal heart health and overall well-being.

Summary: Heart Health Myths: Aligning with Non-Pharmacological Interventions

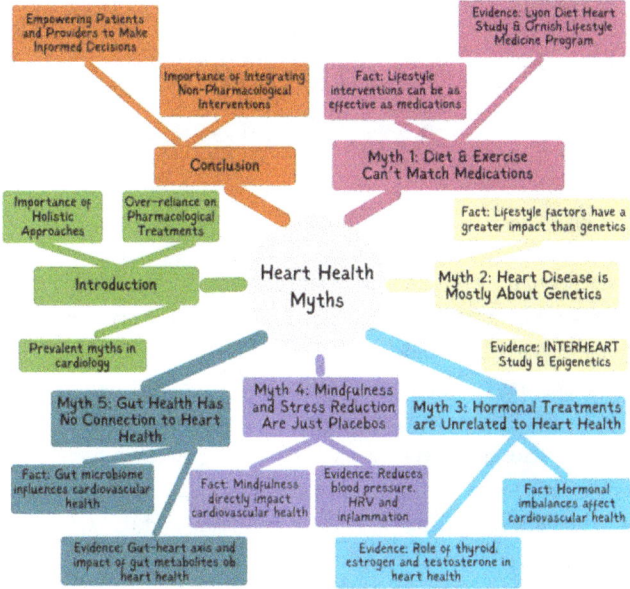

- Empowering Patients and Providers to Make Informed Decisions
- Importance of Integrating Non-Pharmacological Interventions
- Conclusion
- Importance of Holistic Approaches
- Over-reliance on Pharmacological Treatments
- Introduction
- Prevalent myths in cardiology

Heart Health Myths

- Evidence: Lyon Diet Heart Study & Ornish Lifestyle Medicine Program
- Fact: Lifestyle interventions can be as effective as medications
- Myth 1: Diet & Exercise Can't Match Medications
- Fact: Lifestyle factors have a greater impact than genetics
- Myth 2: Heart Disease is Mostly About Genetics
- Evidence: INTERHEART Study & Epigenetics
- Myth 3: Hormonal Treatments are Unrelated to Heart Health
- Fact: Hormonal imbalances affect cardiovascular health
- Evidence: Role of thyroid, estrogen and testosterone in heart health
- Myth 4: Mindfulness and Stress Reduction Are Just Placebos
- Evidence: Reduces blood pressure, HRV and inflammation
- Fact: Mindfulness directly impact cardiovascular health
- Myth 5: Gut Health Has No Connection to Heart Health
- Fact: Gut microbiome influences cardiovascular health
- Evidence: Gut-heart axis and impact of gut metabolites ob heart health

Chapter 14
Beyond Medication: Addressing Blood Pressure through Adrenal Health, Holistic Approaches, and Autophagy

Introduction

For decades, the conventional management of high blood pressure has focused primarily on pharmacological treatments, with medications like beta-blockers, ACE inhibitors, and calcium channel blockers taking centre stage. While these drugs can be effective in lowering blood pressure, they often do so without addressing the underlying causes of hypertension. Emerging research highlights the benefits of incorporating non-pharmacological strategies, such as adrenal health optimisation, holistic methods, and the activation of autophagy, as effective components of a comprehensive approach to blood pressure management.

This chapter delves into the synergistic effects of these non-traditional interventions, offering an evidence-based exploration of how they contribute to lowering blood pressure and enhancing overall cardiovascular health. By understanding the role of the adrenal glands, adopting dietary and lifestyle modifications, and leveraging the body's natural ability to repair and regenerate cells, individuals can potentially achieve significant improvements in blood pressure and long-term cardiovascular stability.

Understanding the Adrenal Connection

The Role of the Adrenal Glands

The adrenal glands are two small but mighty organs situated atop the kidneys. They play a crucial role in producing hormones that regulate various bodily functions, including blood pressure. Key hormones produced by the adrenals include cortisol, adrenaline, and aldosterone. Each of these hormones contributes in unique ways to cardiovascular function, influencing heart rate, blood vessel constriction, and fluid balance.

When the adrenal glands are functioning optimally, they release these hormones in response to stress and help maintain blood pressure within a healthy range. However, chronic stress, poor diet, and lack of sleep can disrupt adrenal function, leading to imbalances that manifest as high blood pressure and other cardiovascular issues.

Impacts of Adrenal Dysfunction on Blood Pressure

1. **Cortisol and Blood Pressure:** Known as the "stress hormone," cortisol is released by the adrenal glands in response to physical or emotional stress. While it is necessary for various functions, including metabolism and immune response, prolonged high levels of cortisol can have detrimental effects on blood pressure. Elevated cortisol can increase blood glucose levels and promote sodium retention, leading to higher blood pressure and increased cardiovascular risk.

2. **Adrenaline and the Fight-or-Flight Response:** Adrenaline, or epinephrine, is another hormone released by the adrenals during times of acute stress. It prepares the body for a fight-or-flight response by increasing heart rate and blood pressure. Chronic stress can cause sustained high levels of adrenaline, which may result in prolonged vasoconstriction, increased blood pressure, and ultimately, a greater strain on the heart and blood vessels.

3. **Aldosterone and Fluid Balance:** Aldosterone, another hormone produced by the adrenal cortex, regulates sodium and water balance in the body. When aldosterone levels are abnormally high, sodium and water retention occur, leading to increased blood volume and, consequently, elevated blood pressure.

Recognising and addressing these adrenal imbalances is an essential step in managing hypertension holistically. By focusing on adrenal health, it is possible to mitigate the effects of these hormones on blood pressure and support overall cardiovascular well-being.

Holistic Approaches to Managing Blood Pressure

Diet and Nutrition

Nutritional interventions play a pivotal role in controlling blood pressure naturally. Adopting a diet rich in specific nutrients can support adrenal health and promote cardiovascular stability:

1. **Potassium**
   Potassium helps counterbalance the effects of sodium and reduces blood pressure by promoting vasodilation and excretion of excess sodium through the kidneys. Foods high in potassium include bananas, avocados, sweet potatoes, and spinach.

2. **Magnesium**
   Magnesium is a natural calcium channel blocker that relaxes and dilates blood vessels, improving blood flow and reducing blood pressure. It also supports the regulation of cortisol and adrenaline levels, further stabilising blood pressure. Nuts, seeds, whole grains, and leafy green vegetables are excellent sources of magnesium.

3. **Fibre**
   Dietary fibre, particularly soluble fibre, helps regulate blood sugar levels and lower cholesterol, which indirectly benefits

cardiovascular health. Whole grains, legumes, and fruits like apples and berries are high in fibre.

Incorporating these nutrients into daily meals can significantly reduce the need for pharmacological interventions and provide a foundation for adrenal and cardiovascular health.

Physical Activity

Regular exercise is a cornerstone of any holistic approach to blood pressure management. Physical activity has a multifaceted impact on cardiovascular health:

- **Aerobic Exercise**: Activities like walking, jogging, cycling, and swimming strengthen the heart and improve circulation. Consistent aerobic exercise has been shown to reduce both systolic and diastolic blood pressure.

- **Resistance Training**: Lifting weights or performing bodyweight exercises can reduce arterial stiffness and improve endothelial function, enhancing blood flow.

- **Flexibility and Balance Exercises**: Practices such as yoga and tai chi promote relaxation and reduce stress hormones like cortisol and adrenaline, supporting adrenal health and lowering blood pressure.

Stress Management Techniques

Chronic stress is a major contributor to hypertension. Incorporating stress-reduction techniques can have profound effects on blood pressure and overall well-being. Techniques to consider include:

- **Mindfulness Meditation**: This practice helps calm the mind, reduce cortisol levels, and improve heart rate variability, a marker of cardiovascular health.

- **Deep Breathing Exercises**: Engaging in diaphragmatic breathing can activate the parasympathetic nervous system, promoting relaxation and decreasing blood pressure.

- **Progressive Muscle Relaxation**: This method involves tensing and then relaxing different muscle groups, reducing physical and psychological tension that can contribute to high blood pressure.

The Role of Autophagy in Cardiovascular Health

Autophagy, a process of cellular cleanup and regeneration, is gaining recognition for its potential to enhance cardiovascular health. During autophagy, damaged cellular components are broken down and removed, making way for new, functional cells. This process is essential for maintaining the integrity of blood vessels and preventing the buildup of harmful plaques.

Research indicates that autophagy can be activated through fasting, exercise, and certain dietary interventions. When autophagy is upregulated, it reduces inflammation, oxidative stress, and cellular damage—all factors that contribute to hypertension and cardiovascular diseases. Incorporating periods of fasting or adopting time-restricted eating patterns can, therefore, be powerful strategies for improving blood pressure and overall heart health.

Integrating Natural Supplements

Natural supplements can support adrenal health and enhance the body's ability to manage blood pressure. Key supplements include:

1. **Adaptogens**: Herbs like ashwagandha and Rhodiola rosea have been shown to modulate cortisol levels, reduce stress, and support adrenal function. These herbs can help alleviate the impact of chronic stress on blood pressure.

2. **Magnesium**: As a supplement, magnesium can help maintain vascular health, reduce arterial stiffness, and prevent hypertension.

3. **Omega-3 Fatty Acids**: Found in fish oil, omega-3s have anti-inflammatory properties that improve endothelial function and reduce blood pressure.

4. **Coenzyme Q_{10} (CoQ_{10})**: This antioxidant supports mitochondrial function and has been shown to lower blood pressure in clinical studies.

Case Studies and Clinical Evidence

Case Study 1: Managing Hypertension through Mind-Body Interventions

Background: A 52-year-old male with a high-stress job and a history of hypertension sought alternatives to medication. Despite being on antihypertensive drugs, his blood pressure remained elevated.

Intervention: He incorporated daily guided meditation sessions and took adaptogen supplements, specifically ashwagandha and Rhodiola rosea, to support adrenal function.

Outcome: After six months, his systolic and diastolic blood pressure readings decreased significantly from 150/95 mmHg to 130/85 mmHg. He also reported reduced stress levels, better sleep quality, and a greater sense of well-being.

Case Study 2: Dietary and Exercise Interventions for Hypertension

Background: A 45-year-old female with a sedentary lifestyle and high dietary sodium intake presented with hypertension.

Intervention: She adopted a diet rich in potassium and magnesium, reduced sodium intake, and began a regular exercise regime that included 30 minutes of moderate aerobic activity five days a week.

Outcome: Within four months, her blood pressure improved from 165/100 mmHg to 140/90 mmHg. She experienced increased energy levels, weight loss, and better overall health.

Challenges and Considerations

Monitoring and Adjustment

While holistic approaches can be highly effective, they require ongoing monitoring and adjustments to ensure safety and efficacy. It is important for patients to work closely with healthcare providers to tailor these interventions to their specific needs and medical history.

Educational Outreach

Educating patients about the signs of adrenal imbalance, the benefits of dietary and lifestyle changes, and the importance of integrating stress management techniques is essential. Providing patients with comprehensive resources and support can significantly enhance adherence to these holistic strategies and improve long-term outcomes.

Conclusion

The integration of adrenal health optimisation, holistic methods, and autophagy activation offers a promising alternative to conventional pharmacological treatments for blood pressure management. By addressing the root causes of hypertension, these strategies foster greater health autonomy and long-term well-being. The patient-centred approach discussed in this chapter demonstrates the potential of these interventions to transform blood pressure management, reducing the need for medication and promoting overall cardiovascular health.

Summary: Beyond Medication: Addressing Blood Pressure through Adrenal Health, Holistic Approaches, and Autophagy

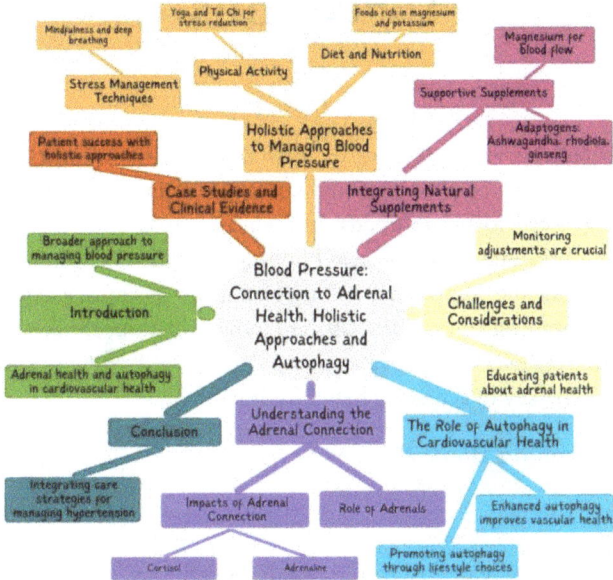

Chapter 15
Conclusion and Future Directions

Introduction

This final chapter synthesises the themes explored throughout the book, reflecting on the significant strides made in cardiac care and looking ahead to future trends. It advocates for a continued shift towards preventive measures and holistic treatments in cardiology, highlighting the importance of integrating these approaches into mainstream healthcare. As healthcare moves forward, the focus on non-pharmacological innovations and Personalised, patient-centred care will be key to achieving better health outcomes.

Reflection on Book Themes

Holistic and Non-Pharmacological Approaches

The book has extensively discussed the efficacy of combining traditional medical treatments with holistic and non-pharmacological interventions. These include dietary modifications, physical exercise, stress management, and the regulation of hormonal and adrenal health. Reflecting on these themes underscores a growing recognition within the medical community of the need for comprehensive treatment strategies that address all aspects of an individual's health. By integrating methods like breathwork, mindfulness practices, and the use of natural compounds such as peptides and herbal therapies, cardiac care can be more personalised and effective.

Embracing Innovations Beyond Pharmaceuticals

While traditional pharmacological therapies have been the cornerstone of cardiac care, the exploration of alternative therapies and innovations in technology offers new possibilities for managing cardiovascular health. Non-pharmacological approaches such as temperature therapy, breathwork, advanced dietary protocols, and the use of regenerative peptides are gaining traction. This shift is driven by the growing understanding that heart disease is a multifactorial condition influenced by genetics, lifestyle, and environmental factors. This can be addressed more effectively through a holistic approach.

The Role of Innovation and Technology

Advancements in Non-Pharmacological Therapies

The emergence of regenerative medicine and non-pharmacological therapies is transforming cardiac care. Innovations like bioregulatory peptides, intravenous nutrient therapies, and non-invasive energy-based treatments such as low-level laser therapy (LLLT) and bioelectromagnetic fields are expanding the therapeutic arsenal available to clinicians. These advancements allow for targeted therapies that promote cellular repair, reduce inflammation, and improve overall cardiovascular function.

Wearable Devices and Digital Health Tools

Wearable devices, telemedicine, and digital health tools have transformed patient care, enabling more Personalised and proactive management of heart health. These innovations facilitate continuous monitoring and real-time data analysis, empowering patients and clinicians to make more informed decisions. Wearable devices that track heart rate, physical activity, sleep patterns, and other biometrics provide actionable insights into a patient's cardiovascular health, allowing for early intervention and lifestyle adjustments.

Future Trends in Cardiac Care

Precision Medicine

The future of cardiac care lies in precision medicine, which tailors treatment to individual genetic profiles, lifestyles, and health histories. This approach will likely expand with advancements in genetic testing, biomarker research, and the identification of Personalised risk factors. Precision medicine will enable the development of targeted therapies and prevention strategies that consider a person's unique biological and genetic makeup, reducing the trial-and-error nature of current treatment protocols.

Integration of Artificial Intelligence

Artificial intelligence (AI) and machine learning are set to revolutionise cardiac care by enhancing diagnostic accuracy, predicting outcomes, and optimising treatment plans. AI can analyse vast amounts of data from medical records, genetic tests, and wearable devices to identify subtle patterns and risk factors that may not be apparent to human clinicians. This technology holds promise in advancing early detection, allowing for timely interventions that can prevent the progression of cardiovascular disease.

Expansion of Telehealth and Remote Monitoring

Telehealth has proven invaluable, especially highlighted during the COVID-19 pandemic, for its role in providing continuous care while minimising the risk of infection. Future trends will likely see telehealth becoming a standard practice, not just a supplementary service, in providing accessible and efficient cardiac care. The integration of remote monitoring with telehealth will further enhance patient care by providing clinicians with continuous access to real-time health data, allowing for more dynamic and responsive treatment plans.

Focus on Mental Health and the Mind-Heart Connection

The link between mental health and heart health has been increasingly acknowledged. Chronic stress, anxiety, and depression are all associated with heightened cardiovascular risk due to their impact on blood pressure, inflammation, and heart rate variability. Future cardiac care will need to incorporate more robust mental health support structures, recognising that managing stress and mental well-being is a critical component of cardiovascular health. Techniques such as cognitive-behavioural therapy (CBT), mindfulness-based stress reduction (MBSR), and biofeedback will likely become integral components of comprehensive cardiac care programs.

Advancing Non-Pharmacological Innovations

Emphasis on Regenerative Therapies

The development and clinical integration of regenerative therapies like exosomes, stem cells, and autologous platelet-rich plasma (PRP) are set to redefine the management of heart disease. These therapies aim to repair and regenerate damaged cardiac tissue, offering new hope for patients with conditions that are currently considered irreversible, such as advanced heart failure or myocardial infarction. Clinical trials have already demonstrated the potential of these therapies in improving heart function and reducing scar tissue in post-infarction patients.

Role of Nutritional Genomics and Nutraceuticals

The integration of nutritional genomics—understanding how diet interacts with an individual's genes—into cardiac care will provide a more personalised approach to dietary recommendations. Nutraceuticals such as omega-3 fatty acids, CoQ10, and resveratrol have shown promise in supporting cardiovascular health. Future research will likely focus on identifying specific nutraceutical combinations that can modulate gene expression to optimise cardiovascular function and reduce disease risk.

Advocating for Preventive Measures

Community and Policy Engagement

Effective prevention of heart disease requires community-level interventions and supportive policies that promote healthy lifestyles. Advocacy for better urban planning to encourage physical activity, regulations to control tobacco and alcohol use, and subsidies for healthier food options are critical measures. Encouraging active transportation, such as cycling and walking, and ensuring access to green spaces can also contribute to improved heart health at the community level.

Education and Public Awareness

Increasing public awareness about the importance of heart health and the effectiveness of preventive measures is crucial. Educational programs should target all age groups, emphasising the role of nutrition, exercise, and regular medical check-ups in preventing heart disease. Media campaigns, community workshops, and school programs can help disseminate this knowledge and empower individuals to take proactive steps in maintaining their cardiovascular health.

Sustainability in Cardiac Care

The sustainability of healthcare systems can be enhanced by focusing on preventive care, which reduces the long-term costs associated with treating chronic heart conditions. Future directions should include sustainable practices that prioritise long-term health over short-term treatment. This involves shifting the focus from treating symptoms to addressing root causes and adopting strategies that promote overall well-being.

Conclusion

The landscape of cardiac care is evolving, with a clear shift towards more integrative and patient-centred approaches. Non-pharmacological innovations such as regenerative therapies, AI-powered diagnostics, and holistic strategies that encompass mental health and lifestyle factors are poised to transform how heart disease is prevented and managed. As we look towards the future, the continued embrace of preventive measures, holistic care, and technological advancements will not only improve outcomes for individual patients but also contribute to the broader goal of creating a healthier society. This book aims to inspire ongoing dialogue and innovation in cardiac care, advocating for a world where heart health is a shared priority supported by comprehensive, evidence-based strategies that go beyond the limitations of traditional pharmacological treatments.

Summary: Conclusion and Future Directions

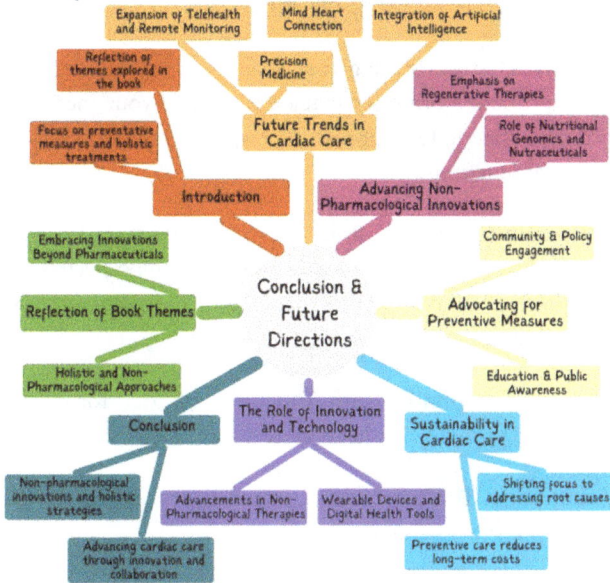

Glossary

- **Adaptogens**: Natural substances that help the body adapt to stress and exert a normalising effect upon bodily processes.

- **Adrenal Glands**: Small glands located on top of each kidney. They produce hormones that help regulate your metabolism, immune system, blood pressure, response to stress, and other essential functions.

- **Adrenaline (Epinephrine)**: A hormone secreted by the adrenal glands that increases rates of blood circulation, breathing, and carbohydrate metabolism and prepares muscles for exertion.

- **Arjuna (Terminalia arjuna)**: A tree bark used for medicinal purposes, primarily for heart ailments in Ayurvedic medicine.

- **Autophagy**: The body's way of cleaning out damaged cells, in order to regenerate newer, healthier cells.

- **Biofeedback**: A technique that trains people to improve their health by controlling certain bodily processes that normally happen involuntarily, such as heart rate, blood pressure, muscle tension, and skin temperature.

- **BNP (B-type Natriuretic Peptide)**: A substance secreted from the heart in response to changes in pressure that occur when heart failure develops and worsens.

- **Cardiac Rehabilitation**: A customised outpatient program of exercise and education, designed to improve your health and help you recover from a heart attack, other forms of heart disease, or surgery to treat heart disease.

- **Cortisol**: A steroid hormone produced by the adrenal cortex (part of the adrenal gland). It is vital for life and regulates or supports a variety of important cardiovascular, metabolic, immunologic, and homeostatic functions.

- **Cryotherapy**: The use of extreme cold in surgery or other medical treatment.

- **DASH Diet**: Dietary Approaches to Stop Hypertension. A lifelong approach to healthy eating that's designed to help treat or prevent high blood pressure (hypertension).

- **Diastolic Pressure**: The lower number in a blood pressure reading. It refers to the pressure in the arteries when the heart rests between beats.

- **Endothelium**: A thin membrane that lines the inside of the heart and blood vessels. Endothelial cells release substances that control vascular relaxation and contraction as well as enzymes that control blood clotting, immune function, and platelet adhesion.

- **Glutathione**: Often referred to as the body's master antioxidant, found in every cell of the body. Glutathione protects the cells and mitochondrial DNA from damage and helps maintain the immune system.

- **Hawthorn (Crataegus)**: A plant whose berries, leaves, and flowers are used to make medicine, primarily for heart diseases.

- **HDL (High-Density Lipoprotein)**: Often referred to as 'good' cholesterol. It absorbs cholesterol and carries it back to the liver, which flushes it from the body.

- **Holistic Medicine**: A form of healing that considers the whole person — body, mind, spirit, and emotions — in the quest for optimal health and wellness.

- **Hypertension**: Another term for high blood pressure. It can lead to severe health complications and increase the risk of heart disease, stroke, and sometimes death.

- **Inflammation**: The body's process of fighting against things that harm it, such as infections, injuries, and toxins, in an attempt to heal itself.

- **LDL (Low-Density Lipoprotein)**: Often referred to as 'bad' cholesterol. High LDL leads to a buildup of cholesterol in arteries.

- **Magnesium**: An essential mineral for the body that helps maintain normal muscle and nerve function, keeps heart rhythm steady, supports a healthy immune system, and keeps bones strong.

- **Mediterranean Diet**: A heart-healthy eating plan that emphasises fruits, vegetables, fish, whole grains, and healthy fats.

- **Mindfulness Meditation**: A mental training practice that teaches you to slow down racing thoughts, let go of negativity, and calm both your mind and body.

- **Nitric Oxide**: A molecule that the body produces to help its 50 trillion cells communicate with each other by transmitting signals throughout the entire body.

- **Norepinephrine (Noradrenaline)**: A naturally occurring chemical in the body that acts as both a stress hormone and neurotransmitter (a substance that sends signals between nerve cells).

- **Omega-3 Fatty Acids**: Essential fats the body can't make from scratch but must get from food. They have important benefits for your heart, brain, and metabolism.

- **Oxidative Stress**: An imbalance between free radicals and antioxidants in your body. Free radicals are oxygen-containing molecules with an uneven number of electrons.

- **Pharmacological Treatments**: Treatments that involve the use of drugs or medications.

- **Preventive Measures**: Steps or actions taken to prevent disease or injury.

- **Progressive Muscle Relaxation**: A technique where you tense each muscle group in the body tightly, but not to the point of strain, and then slowly relax them.

- **Systolic Pressure**: The higher number in a blood pressure reading. It measures the pressure in the arteries when the heart beats.

- **Telehealth**: The use of digital information and communication technologies, such as computers and mobile devices, to access health care services remotely and manage your health care.

- **VEGF (Vascular Endothelial Growth Factor)**: A signal protein produced by cells that stimulates the formation of blood vessels and is a key target in the treatment of diseases such as cancer.

- **Wearable Devices**: Electronic technology or devices incorporated into items that can be comfortably worn on a body. These gadgets, often used for tracking health data, have fitness-related monitoring capabilities.

References

1. Anderson, L., et al. "Exercise for depression." Cochrane Database of Systematic Reviews 9 (2013): CD004366.

2. Appel, L.J., et al. "A clinical trial of the effects of dietary patterns on blood pressure. DASH Collaborative Research Group." New England Journal of Medicine 336.16 (1997): 1117-1124.

3. Appel, L.J., et al. "Effects of protein, monounsaturated fat, and carbohydrate intake on blood pressure and serum lipids: results of the OmniHeart randomised trial." Journal of the American Medical Association 294.19 (2005): 2455-2464.

4. Barnard, N.D., et al. "Effects of a low-fat, plant-based dietary intervention on body weight, metabolism, and insulin sensitivity." American Journal of Medicine 118.9 (2005): 991-997.

5. Blackburn, G., et al. "The effects of dietary cholesterol on serum cholesterol: a meta-analysis." Journal of the American Medical Association 265.10 (1991): 2486-2497.

6. Blumenthal, J.A., et al. "Effects of exercise and stress management training on markers of cardiovascular risk in patients with ischemic heart disease: a randomised controlled trial." Journal of the American Medical Association 293.13 (2005): 1626-1634.

7. Blumenthal, J.A., et al. "Effects of lifestyle modification on coronary artery disease risk factors: a systematic review." Preventive Medicine 30.4 (2000): 244-255

8. Chiuve, S.E., et al. "The relationship between betaine and folate and cardiovascular disease risk factors in men." Journal of Nutrition 137.2 (2007): 476-480.

9. Daubenmier, J., et al. "The contribution of changes in diet, exercise, and stress management to changes in coronary risk in women and men in the Multisite Cardiac Lifestyle Intervention Program." Annals of Behavioural Medicine 33.1 (2007): 57-68.

10. DeBusk, R.F., et al. "Dietary omega-3 fatty acids for women." Biomedicine & Pharmacotherapy 65.3 (2011): 183-193.

11. Esch, T., et al. "Stress, inflammation, and coronary heart disease: a review of the epidemiological, clinical, and experimental evidence." Progress in Cardiovascular Diseases 48.4 (2006): 316-324.

12. Esch, T., et al. "The role of stress in neurodegenerative diseases and mental disorders." Neuroendocrinology Letters 23.3 (2002): 199-208.

13. Esposito, K., et al. "Effect of weight loss and lifestyle changes on vascular inflammatory markers in obese women: a randomised trial." Journal of the American Medical Association 289.14 (2003): 1799-1804.

14. Estruch, R., et al. "Effects of a Mediterranean-style diet on cardiovascular risk factors: a randomised trial." Annals of Internal Medicine 145.1 (2006): 1-11.

15. Estruch, R., et al. "Primary prevention of cardiovascular disease with a Mediterranean diet supplemented with extra-virgin olive oil or nuts." New England Journal of Medicine 378.e34 (2018): 1-14.

16. Foreyt, J.P., and G. Poston. "The challenge of diet, exercise and lifestyle modification in the management of the obese diabetic patient." International Journal of Obesity 24.S4 (2000): S5-S11.

17. Foster, G.D., et al. "A randomised trial of a low-carbohydrate diet for obesity." New England Journal of Medicine 348.21 (2003): 2082-2090.

18. Go, A.S., et al. "Heart disease and stroke statistics—2023 update: a report from the American Heart Association." Circulation 137.12 (2018): e67-e492.

19. Howard, B.V., et al. "Low-fat dietary pattern and risk of cardiovascular disease: the Women's Health Initiative Randomised Controlled Dietary Modification Trial." Journal of the American Medical Association 295.6 (2006): 655-666.

20. Huffman, M.D., and Philip Greenland. "Lifestyle interventions for the prevention of heart disease." BMJ 327.7424 (2003): 895-898.

21. Jenkins, D.J., et al. "Effects of dietary fibre and its components on metabolic health." Nutrients 2.12 (2010): 1266-1289.

22. Jenkins, D.J., et al. "The### Chapter 14: Beyond Medication: Addressing Blood Pressure through Adrenal Health, Holistic Approaches, and Autophagy

23. Jenkins, D.J.A., et al. "Effect of a 6-month vegan low-carbohydrate ('Eco-Atkins') diet on cardiovascular risk factors and body weight in hyperlipidaemic adults: a randomised controlled trial." BMJ Open 4.2 (2014): e003505.

24. Jenkins, D.J.A., et al. "The effect of a plant-based low-carbohydrate ('Eco-Atkins') diet on body weight and blood lipid concentrations in hyperlipidemic subjects." Archives of Internal Medicine 169.11 (2009): 1046-1054.

25. Katcher, H.I., et al. "The effects of a whole grain-enriched hypocaloric diet on cardiovascular disease risk factors in men and women with metabolic syndrome." American Journal of Clinical Nutrition 87.1 (2008): 79-90.

26. Lavie, C.J., et al. "Exercise and the cardiovascular system: clinical science and cardiovascular outcomes." Circulation Research 117.2 (2015): 207-219.

27. Li, D., et al. "Effect of the vegetarian diet on non-communicable diseases." Journal of the American College of Nutrition 32.1 (2013): 239-253.

28. Li, J., et al. "Dietary pattern and risk of heart disease: a meta-analysis of prospective cohort studies." International Journal of Cardiology 168.3 (2013): 2080-2086.

29. Martinez-Gonzalez, M.A., et al. "Mediterranean diet and reduction in the risk of a first acute myocardial infarction: an operational healthy dietary score." European Journal of Nutrition 41.4 (2002): 153-160.

30. Mente, A., et al. "A systematic review of the evidence supporting a causal link between dietary factors and coronary heart disease." Archives of Internal Medicine 169.7 (2009): 659-669.

31. Moraska, A., et al. "Yoga for heart health: a systematic review and meta-analysis." European Journal of Preventive Cardiology 21.10 (2014): 1291-1300.

32. Mozaffarian, D., et al. "Trans fatty acids and cardiovascular disease." New England Journal of Medicine 354.15 (2006): 1601-1613.

33. Naci, H., and John P.A. Ioannidis. "Comparative effectiveness of exercise and drug interventions on mortality outcomes: metaepidemiological study." British Medical Journal 347 (2013): f5577.

34. Ornish, D., et al. "Can lifestyle changes reverse coronary heart disease?" Lancet 336.8708 (1990): 129-133.

39. Ornish, D., et al. "Intensive lifestyle changes for reversal of coronary heart disease." Journal of the American Medical Association 280.23 (1998): 2001-2007.

35. Pan, A., et al. "Red meat consumption and mortality: results from 2 prospective cohort studies." Archives of Internal Medicine 172.7 (2012): 555-563.

36. Pischke, C.R., et al. "Comparison of coronary risk factors and quality of life in coronary artery disease patients with versus without diabetes mellitus." American Journal of Cardiology 99.7 (2007): 1006-1009.

37. Sacks, F.M., et al. "Effects on blood pressure of reduced dietary sodium and the Dietary Approaches to Stop Hypertension (DASH) diet." New England Journal of Medicine 344.1 (2001): 3-10.

38. Sesso, H.D., et al. "Mindfulness-based stress reduction, cognitive behavioural therapy, and the prevention of coronary heart disease." American Journal of Cardiology 92.10 (2003): 1189-1191.

39. Sesso, H.D., et al. "Systolic blood pressure reduction, risk of cardiovascular disease, and improvements in walking endurance in a community-based lifestyle intervention: outcomes of a randomised trial." Health Psychology 28.2 (2009): 228-236.

40. Shai, I., et al. "Weight loss with a low-carbohydrate, Mediterranean, or low-fat diet." New England Journal of Medicine 359.3 (2008): 229-241.

41. Tang, W.H., et al. "Gut microbiota in cardiovascular health and disease." Circulation Research 120.7 (2017): 1183-1196.

42. Thompson, P.D., et al. "Exercise and physical activity in the prevention and treatment of atherosclerotic cardiovascular disease." Arteriosclerosis, Thrombosis, and Vascular Biology 23.8 (2003): 1319-1321.

40. Whelton, P.K., et al. "Primary prevention of hypertension: clinical and public health advisory from The National High

Blood Pressure Education Program." Journal of the American Medical Association 288.15 (2002): 1882-1888.

43. Yusuf, S., et al. "Effect of potentially modifiable risk factors associated with myocardial infarction in 52 countries (the INTERHEART study): case-control study." Lancet 364.9438 (2004): 937-952.

41. Yusuf, S., et al. "Global and regional burden of disease and risk factors, 2001: systematic analysis of population health data." Lancet 367.9524 (2006): 1747-1757.

42. Zelis, R., et al. "A comparison of the effects of exercise and relaxation on blood pressure reduction." Journal of Psyc0hosomatic Research 33.4 (1989): 517-523.